CRYSTAL PAIRINGS

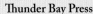

Thunder Bay Press
An imprint of Printers Row Publishing Group
9717 Pacific Heights Blvd, San Diego, CA 92121
www.thunderbaybooks.com • mail@thunderbaybooks.com

Printers Row Publishing Group is a division of Readerlink Distribution Services, LLC.
Thunder Bay Press is a registered trademark of Readerlink Distribution Services, LLC.

Correspondence regarding the content of this book should be sent to Thunder Bay Press, Editorial Department, at the above address. Author, illustration, and rights inquiries should be addressed to Quarto Publishing, The Old Brewery, 6 Blundell St, London, N7 9BH. www.quarto.com

Thunder Bay Press
Publisher   Peter Norton
Associate Publisher   Ana Parker
Editor   Dan Mansfield

Quarto Publishing
Deputy Art Director   Martina Calvio
Assistant Editor   Charlene Fernandes
Copyeditor   Caroline West
Designer   Josse Pickard
Junior Designer   India Minter
Photographer   Nicki Dowey
Publisher   Lorraine Dickey

Library of Congress Control Number: 2022937819

ISBN: 978-1-6672-0161-0

Printed in China

26 25 24 23 22   1 2 3 4 5

CRYSTAL PAIRINGS

POWERFUL CRYSTAL COMBINATIONS FOR WELL-BEING

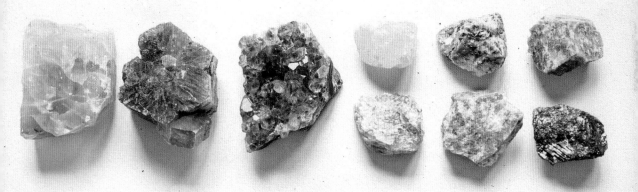

EMILY SUZANNE RAYOW

THUNDER BAY
P · R · E · S · S
San Diego, California

Contents

RUBY
12

GARNET
14

VANADINITE
16

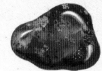

RED CORAL
18

CARNELIAN
20

SUNSTONE
22

AMBER
24

PYRITE
26

CITRINE
28

GOLDEN HEALER QUARTZ
30

HONEY CALCITE
32

EMERALD
34

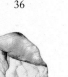

JADE
36

MOLDAVITE
38

MALACHITE
40

CHRYSOPRASE
42

MOSS AGATE
44

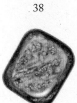

PERIDOT
46

LAPIS LAZULI
48

SAPPHIRE
50

AQUAMARINE
52

TURQUOISE
54

LABRADORITE
56

LARIMAR
58

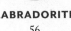

GRANDIDIERITE
60

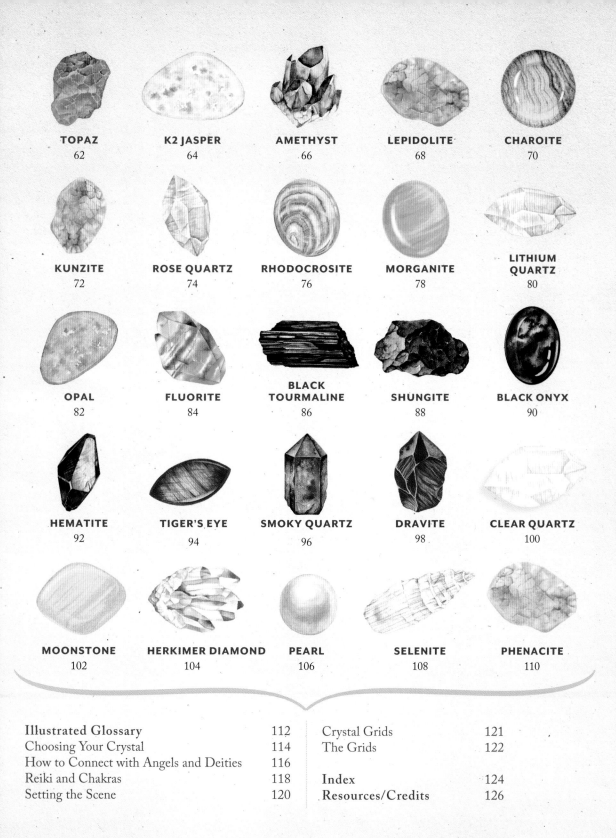

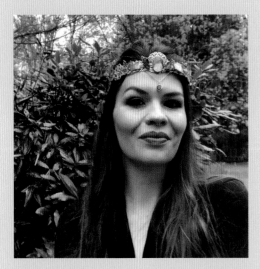

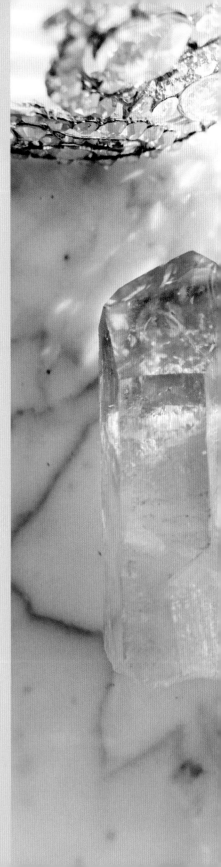

Meet Emily

I do not remember when my love for rocks and crystals began; it feels like something that has always been inside me. When I was in grade school, my father worked at an optometrist's office and brought home a clear, spinning, eyeglass-display case for me to store my tumbled stones and crystal treasures. It came with me to every show-and-tell at school, and some of those stones I still have today.

I always knew I was an artist. When I began to make jewelry, embedding crystal beads into leather cuffs, it set off a spark in my soul. I became reacquainted with my love of rocks from so long ago. I began to teach myself the meanings of crystals alongside developing my jewelry line: working with crystals made my spirit happy.

I attribute my following on social media to the collective desire for self-healing tools and talismans in this age of awakening. I believe crystals and stones are gifts to us from the earth—to bring healing, enlightenment, or simple joy from gazing at something beautiful. With this book, I hope to encourage people to tap into their innate sense of intuition and empowerment.

"WORKING WITH CRYSTALS MADE MY SPIRIT HAPPY."

ABOUT THIS BOOK

Through the ages, crystals have taken on much spiritual significance and have become the focus of many different types of healing techniques, from carrying them in your pocket as a protective amulet to using them in your Reiki or chakra practices.

Directory of Crystals (pages 10-111)

This part features fifty crystals organized by color. Each crystal is explored in depth, from its appearance and rarity to its spiritual healing properties and its use in gridwork. The right-hand panel will tell you which crystals to combine.

Topics discussed: Appearance; Meaning; Rarity; For Your Star Sign; In a Daily Ritual; In Reiki; Angels and Deities; Working with Chakras; For Protection; In a Crystal Grid; Healing Properties; As a Pairing.

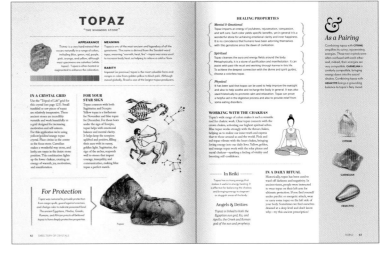

Illustrated Glossary (pages 112-123)

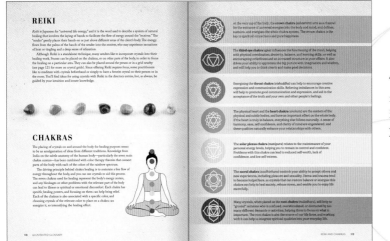

This part explains in detail the topics referenced in the Directory of Crystals, including Reiki, chakras, and choosing your crystal.

Introduction

Just as crystals coexist in harmony in the earth, so too can they be combined in crystal healing. While working with a single stone may bring powerful shifts in your life, "pairing" or grouping stones will often amplify or enhance their effects. Combining stones also allows you to channel healing toward different aspects of a particular issue or to two or more areas of your life that you want to work on simultaneously.

Certain crystal combinations work particularly well together, and I share these and other personal favorites throughout the book. You might also like to choose stones from the same color group, since crystals of similar hues can offer subtle variations on a particular effect. Or you may wish to combine stones that are associated with one of the chakras or a specific area of the body—or perhaps those that encompass a particular quality you wish to cultivate in your life. Crystals from the same family group (such as the quartzes) will always complement each other.

The more you learn about crystals, the easier it becomes to trust your intuition and create your own pairings and groupings. So, while this book looks at my personal findings, know that your own inner wisdom will soon become your guide.

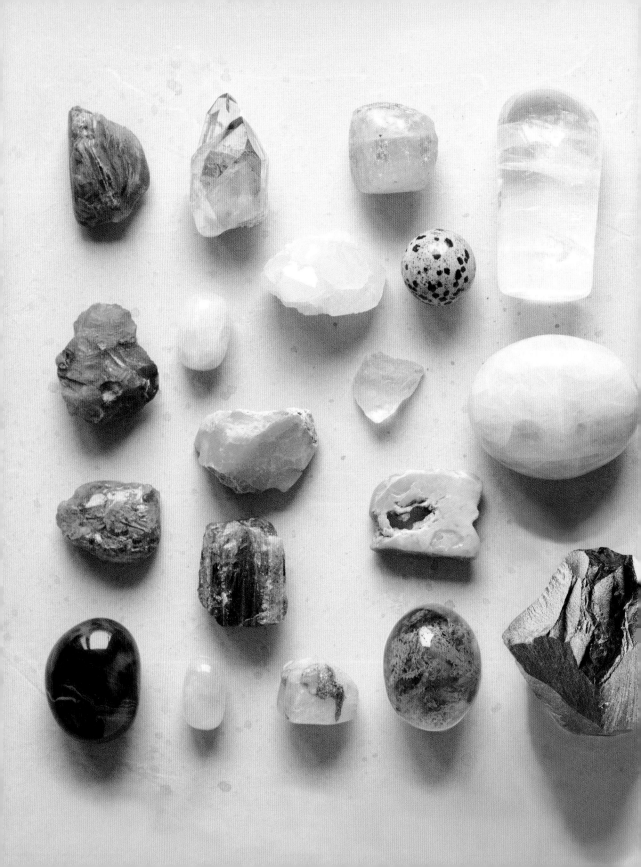

Directory of Crystals

In this directory, you will find fifty beautiful crystals, organized by color to help you find the right stone for you. Each entry offers a fascinating insight into the crystal's energetic properties, how it may support your emotional, physical, and spiritual healing, and the recommended pairings and grids that you can use to enhance its effects.

RUBY

"THE KING OF PRECIOUS STONES"

APPEARANCE

RUBY is the red variety of corundum (when blue in color, it is called sapphire), and gains its coloration from the presence of the mineral chromium. The most valuable specimens are vibrant in color or transparent, although all natural rubies do contain inclusions.

MEANING

Ruby has symbolized nobility, fortune, and passion for thousands of years. In ancient Sanskrit scripture it was referred to as *ratnaraj*, which translates as "king of precious stones."

RARITY

Fine specimens of ruby fetch the highest prices of any colored gem, but lower-quality pieces are available and quite affordable.

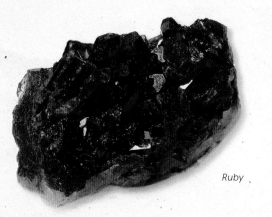

Ruby

For Protection

Many cultures throughout history have associated rubies with protection from harm and evil spirits. The ancient Burmese believed rubies pierced into the flesh would keep warriors safe on the battlefield. They've been thought to bring favor from the gods when used in sacrifice and great power to rulers when worn atop the head or breast.

IN A CRYSTAL GRID

Use the "Vesica Piscis" grid for this crystal (see page 122). Raw, rough rubies work well; you don't need high-quality or faceted gems. Harness the power of the corundum family by pairing ruby with blue sapphire to create a grid for calm and balance. Ruby has a fiery energy that balances well with sapphire's cooling wind energy. Use a clear quartz as the focus stone and ruby and sapphire as the way and desire stones, as you see fit.

WORKING WITH THE CHAKRAS

Both the root chakra and the heart chakra are strongly affected by the illustrious ruby. Muladhara, the root chakra, is our base for stability, survival, and sexuality, as symbolized by the color red. It hums with life-force energy and when it is imbalanced, all other chakras will be affected. Anahata, the chakra of the heart, also resonates with the energy of the ruby crystal, particularly when it is more pink in color. Ruby is a wonderful tool for working through painful trauma (root chakra) and learning to open yourself again to new experiences (heart chakra).

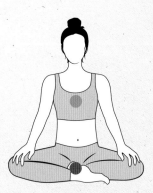

FOR YOUR STAR SIGN

Ruby is the traditional birthstone for the month of July and the star sign of Cancer. The fiery color of this stone speaks to the heat of the season and the passionate personalities of those born under this zodiacal sign. Cancers are loyal, emotional, and intuitive—a perfect match for their crystal counterpart. Ruby helps to keep this water sign grounded and emotionally secure, so that they can flourish and openly share their generous heart with the world.

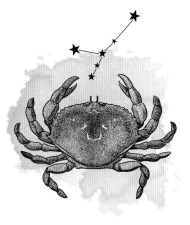

IN A DAILY RITUAL

Ancient civilizations would embed rubies in the foundations of buildings to fill the space with energies of protection, good fortune, and abundance. Throw it back to ancient times by placing a few rough ruby stones in the ground around your home or even just in the four corners of a room. See if you notice a positive change in the energy around you!

Angels & Deities

Ancient Hindus believed rubies the most precious of gems, and would leave them as offerings to the god Krishna.

—— In Reiki ——

Ruby is a strong stimulator of energy flow, particularly in the root chakra region. Place close to the pelvic area, either on or around the body, to activate energy.

HEALING PROPERTIES

Mental & Emotional
Ruby has long been associated with love, passion, and vitality. It is intensely healing for the heart and emotional body. Use ruby to renew feelings of optimism or excitement about life. Ruby can also help rekindle feelings of desire and passion in a relationship that may feel a little stale.

Spiritual
Ruby connects us to the very energy of love and, most importantly, to the amazing power of divine love. It brings a spark and sense of awakening to the spirit. If you are someone who is searching for your true, spiritual purpose in life, simply allow ruby to guide you on your way.

Physical
Unsurprisingly, rubies connect with the heart and the blood. Circulation issues, menstruation, and blood disorders all fall within the realm of ruby. It can also be used for reproductive issues and a healthy pregnancy, as well as overall physical vitality.

& As a Pairing

When ruby is paired with the power of **SHUNGITE**, it creates an unbeatable duo of protective energy; fiery ruby amplifies shungite's energetic shielding abilities. Ruby also harmonizes with the energy of **BLUE SAPPHIRE**, its crystal cousin. The ruby grounds and connects through the lower chakras, while blue sapphire creates higher chakric connections with spirit. Ruby also makes a powerful and beneficial pairing with richly colored **RED CORAL**.

SHUNGITE

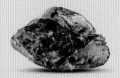

BLUE SAPPHIRE

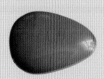

RED CORAL

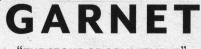

GARNET

"THE STONE OF COMMITMENT"

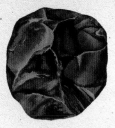

APPEARANCE

GARNET exists in a rainbow of colors: yellow, orange, pink, green, and black, but we associate it most often with a deep burgundy color. It has been used for millennia as jewelry, as well as an abrasive material.

MEANING

The word *garnet* is derived from the Latin *granatum*, which is a reference to the pomegranate seed that it so closely resembles. Garnet was said to be the only source of light on Noah's Ark.

RARITY

Garnet is one of the most abundant minerals on the earth, although some colors—including pink and green—are rarer than others.

FOR YOUR STAR SIGN

Those born in the month of January are lucky to be able to call this juicy gem their birthstone. The Capricorn, as an earth sign, is one of stability and manifestation. Their positive qualities are amplified by working with garnet crystal, which provides grounding and balance. Those born under the sign of the sea-goat are often successful, driven, and brutally honest. What they lack in emotional sensitivity they make up for in pure ambition, but with the help of garnet's loving influence, the edges are softened a little.

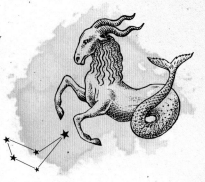

IN A DAILY RITUAL

If you're feeling unmoored, stagnant, or unstable, you might consider some daily work on your root chakra. The practice is simple: sit on the ground, holding a garnet in your right hand. Imagine muladhara, the root chakra located at the base of your spine, and send healing energy to it from the stone in your hand. You may use the scent of patchouli, sandalwood, or vetiver as an accompaniment.

Angels & Deities

Garnet has a connection with the Greek goddess Persephone, who ate the forbidden pomegranate fruit and thus split the world into seasons of light and dark.

For Protection

With an almost unrivaled history of human adornment, early Christians, Celts, ancient Egyptians, Muslims, and Native Americans all attributed powers of protection to the glowing garnet. Warriors would wear garnet into battle and travelers carried the gem to safeguard against danger and robbery.

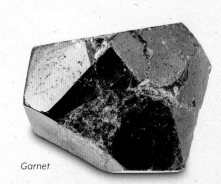

Garnet

WORKING WITH THE CHAKRAS

Most garnets are strong root chakra stones. They bring vitality, spark, rejuvenation—activating *prana*, or life-force energy. The effects of this gem are not subtle: when working with garnet, expect intense shifts. It can activate *kundalini* energy, the coil of divine energy located at the base of the spine, which connects us to our truest essence. Tsavorite, the green garnet, is an excellent heart chakra opener, bringing an electricity and healing light to the emotional body. Spessartine garnet, in its orange and golden hues, works with the sacral and solar plexus chakras.

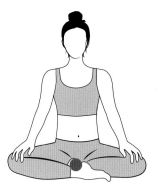

IN A CRYSTAL GRID

Use the "Seed of Life" grid for this crystal (see page 122). Tap into garnet's history as a stone of devotion by creating a grid for your romantic relationship. Place a piece of rose quartz in the focus stone position. Garnet fits beautifully into the way stone position, helping us achieve a fulfilling relationship through passion, commitment, and trust. Finish with green calcite as the desire stones and accent with a personal touch: a ring, photograph, petals, or your beloved's name written on a piece of paper.

— In Reiki —

Apply garnet anywhere there seems to be a shortage or stagnation of energy. Use that spark of fire to invigorate any chakric, emotional, or physical problem area. It is particularly useful in the root chakra, for the lower back/pelvic area.

HEALING PROPERTIES

Mental & Emotional
Garnet has long been known as a stone of love, commitment, and passion. It is therefore no coincidence that throughout history it has been described as holding a light, or fire, inside it. This powerful crystal has the unique ability to make us feel both grounded and full of life and energy.

Spiritual
Through its earthly connection, garnet provides us with a feeling of strength and stability—it can be compared to an ethereal, supportive hand resting on our shoulder, affirming that we are safe and loved. This allows us to be the truest form of ourselves: in our work, relationships, and creative endeavors.

Physical
Garnet is said to be able to make a connection with the heart and blood, thus improving the circulatory system. It can also be used to enhance the libido and other areas of sexual dysfunction. Additionally, you can try calling on the powers of garnet to bring more energy to a sluggish metabolism.

& As a Pairing

Combining **CARNELIAN** with garnet brings intense power and energy to the lower chakras, from root to sacral to solar plexus. This infuses our life with a sense of self-confidence, motivation, and passion. If you're seeking to enhance garnet's more amorous attributes, pair it with **GREEN CALCITE** or any heart chakra stones.

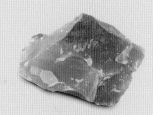

CARNELIAN

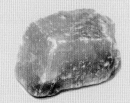

GREEN CALCITE

VANADINITE

"THE STONE OF VITALITY"

APPEARANCE

VANADINITE is a hexagonal, reddish-orange form of apatite crystal. It is formed from oxidized lead ore, and made up of lead, vanadium, oxygen, and chlorine. It is known for its fiery coloration and attractive crystal structures.

MEANING

Vanadinite imparts a sense of adventure, passion, and motivation. It helps writers and artists to tap into deep inspiration and move through any kind of creative block.

RARITY

Vanadinite is an uncommon mineral, but some recent discoveries in Morocco have made it more obtainable for the general collector.

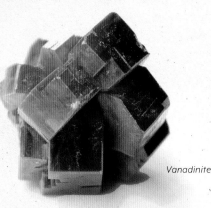

Vanadinite

For Protection

Known as a powerful protector against EMF radiation, vanadinite makes a good addition to any workspace. Due to its ability to ground into the earth, vanadinite has an energizing and detoxifying effect on the chakric system and energy field of the body.

IN A CRYSTAL GRID

Use the "Metatron's Cube" grid for this crystal (see page 123). Creating a grid with vanadinite is a real treat. This grid is well suited to aligning with a professional or creative project. If you find yourself in the midst of such an undertaking and need a little extra "push," try the following. Using the grid template, use a large quartz crystal cluster as the focus stone. Use six small pieces of vanadinite in the way stone position and six pieces of carnelian in the desire stone position. This recipe asks the universe for the fortitude to see your project through to the end, with passion and confidence.

WORKING WITH THE CHAKRAS

The sacral chakra, svadhisthana, is most aligned with vanadinite. This is the energy center for sexuality, vitality, creativity, and drive. However, all three lower chakras (root, sacral, and solar plexus) are affected by this powerful crystal. These chakras are often blocked by deep, unresolved fears. The collective result of a balanced, healthy lower set of chakras is a deeper sense of self and purpose, heightened motivation and lust for life, increased self-confidence, and thus healthier relationships with others. This is the foundation upon which all higher-vibrational spiritual work must depend.

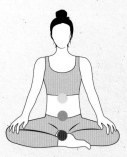

FOR YOUR STAR SIGN

Vanadinite connects with the signs of Aries and Virgo. Aries, a fire sign, is driven, passionate, and persistent. The sign of the ram loves tackling new projects and endeavors. Vanadinite helps the often-impatient Aries see these tasks through to completion. Virgo, on the other hand, is a little more cautious and analytical and capitalizes on vanadinite's fiery, driving-force energy. The already organized Virgoan personality creates an unbeatable force when combined with vanadinite's methodical energy.

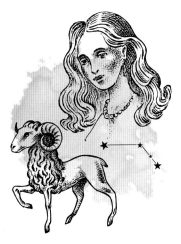

IN A DAILY RITUAL

Placing a piece of vanadinite under your pillow at night is a great way to wake up energized and ready to tackle the day! It's the crystal-energy version of a double shot of espresso. This takes the place of many hands-on crystal meditations and rituals, as it's best not to handle vanadinite for prolonged periods of time.

Angels & Deities

Named after the Norse goddess of fertility and beauty, Vanadis (also known as Freyja).

—— In Reiki ——

Creating a grid around the body—avoiding direct contact with the skin—is advised, specifically around the lower chakras. From the root chakra (pelvic) region up to the solar plexus (navel) region, vanadinite's energies are very effective.

HEALING PROPERTIES

Mental & Emotional
Vanadinite is all about the mental process: helping with clarity, focus, and organization. It combats fatigue, keeping you energized and motivated. Turn to this red gem if you want to rekindle desire and passion in a romantic relationship, your professional life, or any kind of creative endeavor.

Spiritual
Vanadinite has a very grounding vibration and can be useful in connecting to earth energy. This is especially helpful when you spend a lot of time in meditation or enjoying other forms of spiritual journeying. Vanadinite helps us to access deep intuition and inspiration, and also assists us to manifest those things into our daily lives.

Physical
Vanadinite is useful for soothing all kinds of respiratory issues, such as asthma, bronchitis, chronic breathing problems, and more. It can also be used to counter the effects of aging. Anyone who suffers from chronic fatigue will find an ally in this red gem, but avoid keeping it in direct contact with the skin as the lead content can be toxic.

& As a Pairing

To enhance the sacral chakra-stoking qualities of this fiery crystal, combine it with **CARNELIAN**. The total effect of these two driving, passionate stones is greater than the sum of their parts. For a calming effect, or to temper the intense energies of vanadinite, combine with its mineral cousin, **BLUE APATITE**.

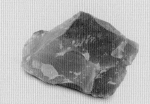

CARNELIAN

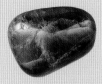

BLUE APATITE

RED CORAL

"THE GEMSTONE OF LIFE-FORCE ENERGY"

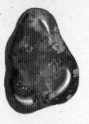

APPEARANCE

RED CORAL, also known as precious coral, is not technically a crystal at all. Instead, it is an "organic gemstone" that is composed of the skeletal remains of marine polyps built up over millions of years. Red coral can be pink, orange, or red in color.

MEANING

Ancient Egyptian, Celtic, Hindu, and Islamic cultures all prized red coral very highly. Literally the product of lifetimes of growth, red coral represents lifeblood, vitality, wisdom, and strength.

RARITY

The most valuable varieties are a deep blood-red and come from the Mediterranean Sea. Source from responsible dealers or vintage dealers to help combat overharvesting.

IN A DAILY RITUAL

Red coral is considered sacred in traditional Hindu culture and astrology. It is known as the "moonga stone," and there are very specific instructions for how you should work with it. It is recommended that you wear red coral on a Tuesday (the day of Mars), after cleansing it with incense and a mantra. Tradition also teaches that you should wear red coral with a gold, rose gold, or copper color.

FOR YOUR STAR SIGN

Red coral has always been connected to the planet Mars, which governs energy, passion, and assertiveness. Mars rules over both the signs of Aries and Scorpio, making red coral their perfect crystal companion. Aries, the sign of the ram, is playful and adventurous and red coral will embolden these endearing qualities. Scorpio has similarly fiery qualities, but can use some tempering from time to time, so should make use of the grounding qualities of red coral.

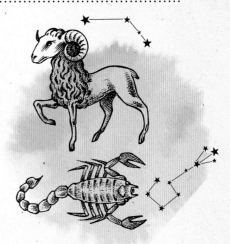

WORKING WITH THE CHAKRAS

Red coral is predominantly a root chakra stone. The first chakra, muladhara, located at the base of the spine, is responsible for our survival instinct, sense of stability, and basic emotional needs. It is no coincidence that this chakra is first in the series of energy centers running throughout the body because unless these needs are met, all other pursuits are rendered null and void. Red coral, with its bold color and assertive energy, helps to strengthen muladhara, instilling in us a primal sense of security and confidence in who we are.

Angels & Deities

In Greek mythology, red coral was said to have formed from Medusa's blood when her head was severed by Perseus.

— In Reiki —

Place pieces of red coral around the pelvic region during Reiki sessions to stimulate the root chakra and bring balance to the hips, pelvis, reproductive organs, and lower digestive tract.

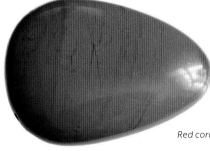
Red coral

For Protection

In AD 77, Pliny the Elder described red coral as having the power to protect against danger. It was thought to ward off magic spells and dark energies. Spiritualists and psychic mediums still use red coral when traveling between realms, to provide safety and a shield of protection.

IN A CRYSTAL GRID

Use the "Square" grid for this crystal (see page 123). If you suspect you may have an imbalanced root chakra, creating a crystal grid to send energy to muladhara is an effective practice. Signs of an improperly functioning root chakra include feelings of fearfulness or insecurity, low self-esteem, or issues with the sexual organs. To create this healing grid, use smoky quartz as your focus stone, surrounded by pieces of red jasper as way stones and red coral as desire stones. This combination of stones is a recipe for increased vitality, strength, security, and confidence.

HEALING PROPERTIES

Mental & Emotional
Red coral imparts a sense of life-force energy, perseverance, and transformation. It can help to shift you out of a slump or depression, or bring an infusion of fresh energy to a situation. Use this maritime marvel if you want to increase your libido, feel a sense of playfulness, and enjoy a general lust for life.

Spiritual
Red coral grounds us in our earthly bodies, which helps us to feel secure and protected. It is necessary to establish this before we can venture into any higher realms of spirituality. Red coral can also be a very helpful meditation tool, driving away negative energy while allowing the mind's eye to focus and expand.

Physical
In ancient times, red coral was ground into a powder and then taken as a tonic in order to cure a whole array of ailments. It has long since been believed to help with the circulation, issues with the blood, the skeletal system, and skin problems. Historically red coral has even been used to prevent miscarriage, though this has not been proven.

& As a Pairing

RUBY makes a very powerful, beneficial pairing with red coral. The two impart similar energies of renewal, vitality, and passion—and so amplify the other's effects. For root chakra healing, combine with other red or dark-colored stones, like **SMOKY QUARTZ**. Also, pair red coral with its nautical cousin, **PEARL**, to bring an energy of balance.

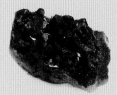

RUBY

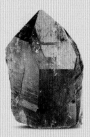

SMOKY QUARTZ

PEARL

CARNELIAN

"THE SUNSET STONE"

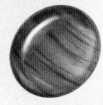

APPEARANCE

CARNELIAN can range from a deep brownish-red to yellow-orange in color. It is a variety of chalcedony, in the quartz crystal family. The ancient Egyptians called carnelian the "sunset stone" due to its bright, fiery appearance.

MEANING

Carnelian symbolizes warmth, vitality, creativity, and joy. The word is derived from the Latin *carneus*, meaning "flesh." It has been worn for millennia to provide protection and revitalization.

RARITY

This semi-precious gemstone is readily available and affordable. It is most often found in bead, cabochon, or tumbled form.

WORKING WITH THE CHAKRAS

Carnelian can be beneficial for all three lower chakras—the root, sacral, and solar plexus chakras—but the sacral chakra in particular responds to this fiery gem. Svadhishthana, the second chakra, which is located just below the navel, is the center of life-force energy, sexuality, and creativity. When this chakra is blocked or imbalanced, you might experience feelings of lethargy, a lack of desire/drive, sexual dysfunction, or compulsive behavior. To balance your sacral chakra, wear or carry carnelian every day, surround yourself with the color orange, spend time near bodies of water when possible, and practice hip-opening yoga poses.

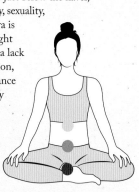

IN A DAILY RITUAL

Carnelian is transformative yet approachable, making it a perfect tool for both novice and experienced crystal workers. There are myriad ways to work with carnelian, and one of the best (and easiest!) is to create a crystal elixir. This is such a fun way to literally infuse your body with healing crystal energy. Simply place a crystal in a glass of drinking water, then let it sit for a few hours before removing the crystal and drinking the infused water.

—— In Reiki ——

Use carnelian if you are suffering from sexual dysfunction or PMS. Combine with other stones that resonate with the lower chakras; smoky quartz is a good choice. Place carnelian on the lower abdomen area for body layout work.

For Protection

You would be hard-pressed to find a stone that more universally represents protection. Spanning millennia and cultures, including ancient Greeks and Romans, Tibetan Buddhists, Muslims, and early Christians, carnelian has always signified safety. It is known as the "Mecca stone" by Muslims, and the Prophet Muhammad supposedly wore a carnelian ring to ensure he had a blessed life after death.

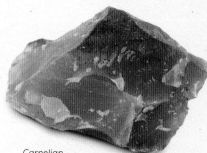

Carnelian

IN A CRYSTAL GRID

Use the "Flower of Life" grid for this crystal (see page 122). All quartz crystals are compatible in a grid, so this is a great foundation if you're unsure of how or where to start. This simple, quartz-based grid uses carnelian, clear quartz, and citrine. It can be a mood booster, increase self-confidence, or be tailored to more specific needs. Use clear quartz as the focus stone, create an inner ring of carnelian as the way stones, and finish with an outer ring of citrine desire stones.

Angels & Deities

The Egyptian goddess Isis was said to use carnelian to protect the souls of the dead. The Bible describes how it was used in the breastplate of Aaron.

HEALING PROPERTIES

Mental & Emotional
Much like its Egyptian name, the "sunset stone," carnelian burns away what is no longer needed and allows us to welcome the new day. It is a crystal of renewed vigor; a stone to assist us in choosing life. It has been used throughout human history by orators for boldness, by warriors for strength, and by lovers for fertility.

Spiritual
Believed by ancient Egyptians to help protect souls on their journey to the afterlife, carnelian has always held the energy of transition. From one life to the next, from one season of life to another—like the fiery fall leaves ushering in winter's bite—carnelian lets us move forward on our path with grace and strength.

Physical
Carnelian is a stone of life-force energy (*chi* in Chinese and *prana* in Sanskrit). Its high iron content creates a strong connection to the bloodstream and it can be used for problems with blood pressure or circulation. In women, it can assist in menstruation and menopause. For men, it can be useful for issues with libido or impotency.

FOR YOUR STAR SIGN

Although carnelian is not a modern birthstone, it is often associated with the late summer and fall months, and the sign of Virgo. The virgin is the only astrological sign depicted by a woman, and Virgos are characterized by their wisdom, loyalty, and logic. Working with carnelian crystals will support the passionate nature of Virgo, while keeping them focused and motivated. It can become a powerful tool for manifestation. Just like the turning of the leaves in this part of the year, carnelian is a symbol of transformation.

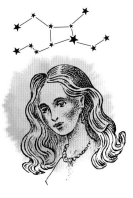

& As a Pairing

Carnelian works well with all varieties of quartz, especially **CITRINE**. Combining it with **ORANGE CALCITE** will enhance the energies of both. **GARNET** and **VANADINITE** also combine beautifully with carnelian in areas of sensuality and vitality. Try pairing carnelian with **RHODOCHROSITE** to help open the heart chakra or with **TOPAZ** to bring energy down to the sacral chakra.

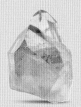

CITRINE

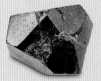

GARNET

VANADINITE

SUNSTONE

"THE SUNSHINE STONE"

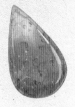

APPEARANCE

Sunstone is a peach/golden-colored variety of feldspar mineral, characterized by a glinting, metallic sheen due to copper, hematite, or goethite inclusions. The optical effect of these light-reflecting inclusions is called aventurescence (or "schiller")—only a few minerals exhibit it.

MEANING

Once used as a primitive compass by the Vikings in order to find their way when navigating, sunstone has the wonderful ability to direct us back to the warmest and most joyful parts of ourselves.

RARITY

Rarer varieties of sunstone, such as transparent pieces from Oregon, fetch high prices, but in general it can be acquired rather easily.

HEALING PROPERTIES

Mental & Emotional

Many ancient cultures had a relationship with sunstone in ritual and lore. Almost always tied to deities of the sun, it has represented energy, vitality, and leadership across millennia. Sunstone can be used to increase your levels of confidence and positivity, as well as combat seasonal depression.

Spiritual

Sunstone is all about the quality of light: warmth, growth, abundance, clarity, and illumination. Its energy represents the divine masculine—that is, assertiveness and strength. Use sunstone to embolden yourself in times of uncertainty or to bring joy back into your life when you have lost sight of the light.

Physical

Sunstone has a very beneficial effect on the process of digestion and metabolism, and can help us to absorb all the available nutrients from what we put into our bodies. It can also be effective in soothing health problems such stomach ulcers, cramps, rheumatism, or arthritis.

For Protection

Sunstone is thought to repel negative energy and so has been used as a protective talisman since ancient times. As a strengthener of intuition and confidence, it empowers us to keep ourselves out of vulnerable situations. As as symbol of the sun and life-force energy, trust sunstone to keep you free from shadow.

—— In Reiki ——

Use sunstone around the second and third (sacral and solar plexus) chakras. Creating a crystal grid around this area of the body can amplify the healing effects.

Angels & Deities

Sunstone is connected to the Egyptian sun god Ra and the Greek god of the sun, Helios.

Sunstone

IN A CRYSTAL GRID

Use the "Flower of Life" grid for this crystal (see page 122). Use sunstone with other vibrant, fiery, energizing crystals to create a grid designed to spark joy in your daily life. Create the grid somewhere you will pass by frequently throughout the day. A citrine tower or cluster makes a perfect focus stone, surrounded by tumbled sunstone and amber pieces. These can be used interchangeably in the way and desire stone positions; use your intuition! You want this grid to spark happiness, so include anything that brings you joy: dried flowers, feathers, beads, and so on—just listen to your heart.

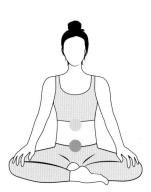

WORKING WITH THE CHAKRAS

With its warm, golden tones, sunstone connects with both the sacral and solar plexus chakras. The sacral chakra, svadhisthana, is the center of our emotions, pleasure, sensuality, and creativity; it is associated with the color orange. A blocked sacral chakra can result in unhealthy relationships, sexual dysfunction, depression, or more. The function of the sacral chakra corresponds with that of the solar plexus chakra, and you can use sunstone to open and balance them both. The solar plexus chakra is our center of confidence and personal power, and connected to yellow and golden colors.

IN A DAILY RITUAL

Sunstone, as we've discussed, has a very real and vibrant connection to the energy of the sun itself. If you're feeling low in energy or depressed, particularly by seasonal affective disorder, charge a piece of this stone in the sunlight for several hours. Carry this crystal around with you throughout your day for a little pick-me-up!

FOR YOUR STAR SIGN

Both Libra and Leo have a special connection with this glowing gem. Libra is a peace-loving sign and dislikes confrontation—sometimes at the expense of their own needs. Sunstone helps Librans to advocate for themselves in a calm and assured way. Leo is a fire sign: all warmth and charisma, with a touch of drama. The sign of the lion is a natural-born leader, making sunstone, with its driving-force energy, a perfect companion.

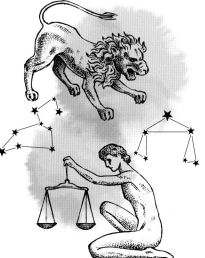

& As a Pairing

Sunstone has a strong, male, yang energy, so pair it with its female yin counterpart, **MOONSTONE**, for a balancing effect on the body, mind, and spirit. Sunstone also resonates strongly with **AMBER** as each is imbued with warm, golden, sunny energy. The crystals in this pairing each exponentially enhance the effects of the other.

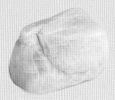

MOONSTONE

AMBER

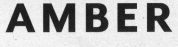

AMBER

"THE STONE OF FROZEN SUNLIGHT"

APPEARANCE
AMBER is fossilized tree resin and falls into the organic gemstone category, usually being between 30 and 130 million years old. Most amber is honey-yellow to orange in color, but it can also be found in shades of white, red, blue, green, or black.

MEANING
Valued since prehistoric times for its beauty and healing properties, amber has always symbolized the sun, warmth, protection, and purification. Beloved across millennia and cultures for its decorative and medicinal purposes.

RARITY
Blue amber, which is a relatively new discovery, is the rarest and most valuable form of amber.

IN A CRYSTAL GRID
Use the "Seed of Life" grid for this crystal (see page 122). A wonderful way to connect with sunny, seasonal energy is to create a grid for the summer solstice. In the Northern Hemisphere, this occurs in June and officially marks the start of summer. To celebrate that bright day, create your grid with a citrine point or cluster as the focus stone, to harness energy from the universe. Surround the citrine with small pieces of amber in the way stone position. For the outer ring, the desire stones, choose pieces of sunstone. Add any natural elements that represent summer to you, such as flower petals and seeds.

FOR YOUR STAR SIGN
Amber, with its myriad healing benefits, can be useful for a number of different astrological signs. The signs most connected with amber, however, are Leo and Aquarius. Fiery, passionate Leo makes a soul connection with this golden gem. It amplifies Leo's most desirable qualities—their confidence, optimism, and creativity. Aquarius will find a comforting ally in amber. It soothes a weary spirit that often occurs in the idealistic and sensitive water-bearer.

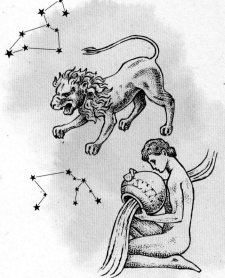

For Protection

Amber has been used through the ages to protect adults and children from disease, the evil eye, and black magic. During the Middle Ages, it was burned for purification. The ancient Egyptians placed amber in burial tombs to protect the souls of the dead in the afterlife.

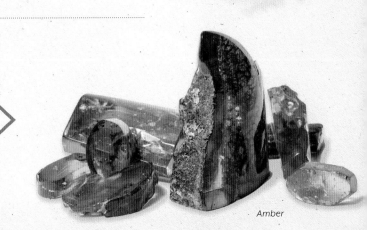

Amber

HEALING PROPERTIES

Mental & Emotional
Amber imbues the wearer with the energy of pure sunlight. Much like a bright, sunny day after a period of gloomy weather, amber reawakens our joy, energy, and motivation. It can assist with depression and moving past grief. The illuminating nature of this organic gem tends to allow our best qualities to shine.

Spiritual
Due to its connection with the natural world and pure life-force energy, amber has an uplifting and purifying effect on the aura. The ancient Chinese believed that when a tiger died, its spirit became this honey-hued gem, so earning it the name "soul of the tiger" and an association with courage and purity.

Physical
Today, amber is most associated with teething necklaces for babies. However, it was once prescribed to ward away the Black Death. Amber can also be effective for alleviating seasonal affective disorder. It has even been thought capable of drawing disease from the body and absorbing pain.

WORKING WITH THE CHAKRAS

Amber is predominantly a stone of the solar plexus chakra, although it can be used for sacral chakra healing as well. The solar plexus, known as *manipura* in Sanskrit (which roughly translates to "city of jewels"), is our center of confidence, self-worth, and emotional balance. It is associated with the element of fire, making it a perfect match for this lively solar stone. Amber represents the meeting of sunlight and earth energy, and wraps us in warm, loving energies—letting us know that we are worthy, capable, and whole.

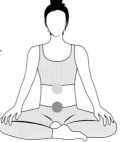

—— In Reiki ——

Amber makes a wonderful tool for hands-on Reiki, as it is actually warm to the touch and brings real comfort and deep healing energy to a session.

Angels & Deities

In Greek mythology, Phaeton (son of Helios, the sun god) was struck down by Zeus. His sisters were turned to trees and their tears became droplets of amber.

IN A DAILY RITUAL
If you want to connect with amber energy, which is essentially the energy of the earth itself, sit with a stone during meditation while burning some copal. Copal is a younger, less ripened form of amber that is harvested and made into incense. Bury the amber in some dirt overnight first if possible, to cleanse the stone and recharge it with earth energy.

& As a Pairing

To amplify its sunny, radiant energies, pair amber with **SUNSTONE** (**PERIDOT** and **HONEY CALCITE** are also complementary). The combined effect of these energies is very helpful for sacral and solar plexus chakra work, or for anyone suffering from seasonal depression. For a deepened earth energy connection, try combining with **MOSS AGATE**.

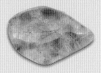

SUNSTONE

PERIDOT

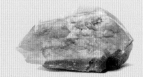

HONEY CALCITE

MOSS AGATE

PYRITE

"THE STONE OF FIRE"

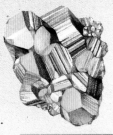

APPEARANCE

Pyrite is also known as "fool's gold" due to its historical tendency to be mistaken for real gold. It often forms in cubic shapes and has a metallic, brassy luster. Pyrite creates sparks when struck against metal and other hard stones.

MEANING

The word *pyrite* is derived from the Greek *pyr*, which means "fire." This striking golden gem certainly lights a fire in the spirit with a strong, masculine energy and it is very protective as a talisman.

RARITY

Pyrite is widely distributed throughout the world. As a result, it is relatively affordable and readily available as specimen stones or in jewelry form.

HEALING PROPERTIES

Mental & Emotional
The effect of pyrite on the emotions is energizing, inspiring, and transformative. Just as fire-ravaged soil feeds new, beautiful growth in plants, so pyrite holds a mirror up to us, so we can eliminate old, toxic traits and behaviors and then reemerge: feeling renewed, revitalized, and transformed.

Spiritual
Pyrite's grounding energy can support us during meditation or spiritual work. It infuses the aura with the energy of abundance, protection, and inspiration. Carry or wear pyrite when you feel you could use an extra "charge" or "sparkle" throughout your day. Let that fiery energy transform the ordinary into extraordinary!

Physical
Pyrite imparts energy and vitality, and can be used to boost your mood. It assists with healthy cellular function and regeneration. This beautiful golden healer is also said to support the digestive, circulatory, and immune systems. Being such a protective stone, it can shield the body against the effects of pollution.

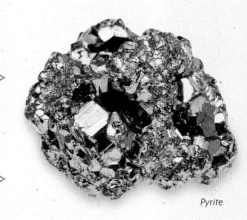

Pyrite

IN A DAILY RITUAL

Pyrite can be a very useful tool when used in feng shui. This is the ancient Chinese practice of arranging and decorating a space in order to bring in desired energies. To work with pyrite according to the rules of feng shui, place a piece in the left-hand corner of your home when you're looking in from the front door. This is the area of the home to work on if you are hoping to enhance your abundance, wealth, and prosperity.

For Protection

One of pyrite's greatest assets is its quality of protection. It connects with fire energy, which is fierce and primal. It is wonderful to wear on the body or place around the home for its shielding vibrations. It also enhances self-confidence, emboldening us to stand up for ourselves and others.

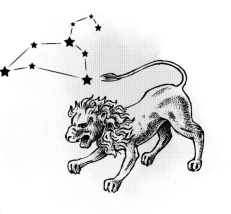

Angels & Deities

Pyrite claims connection with Persephone, queen of the underworld and goddess of spring.

FOR YOUR STAR SIGN

All lions and lionesses born under the sign of Leo may discover that they have a special affinity with this golden gem. Leo is a fire sign, and much like your crystal companion really knows how to get the sparks flying. Dynamic, creative, assertive Leo is grounded by the energy of pyrite. In fact, the energy of pyrite represents Leo's best self: fiery and passionate, yet stable, centered, and self-assured.

WORKING WITH THE CHAKRAS

The solar plexus chakra resonates strongly with pyrite energy. Imagine this chakra as a golden, glowing center of personal power, self-will, and courage. It is represented by the color yellow and the element of fire, making pyrite a natural match for it. When this chakra is imbalanced, you may experience a range of issues, including poor self-esteem, indecisiveness, depression, aggression, or digestive problems. Meditating with a piece of pyrite held over the solar plexus, just above the navel, will help to bring balance to this oh-so-important area.

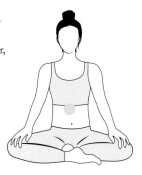

—— In Reiki ——

Pyrite is incredibly effective around the lower chakras: the root, sacral, and solar plexus all benefit from its grounding, invigorating energy. Pyrite can also be used around the female reproductive organs to support them if there are issues.

IN A CRYSTAL GRID

Use the "Spiral" grid for this crystal (see page 122). A grid that almost anyone can benefit from is one designed to bring joy and prosperity into your life. It's so easy to forget about the simple act of inviting more sparkle into our days. Combine pyrite with citrine for a light-filled, positivity-invoking grid designed to uplift the spirit. Use citrine as the focus stone in the grid. Surround the citrine with pyrite in the way stone position. For the desire stones, choose the crystal that brings *you* the most joy! Choose something you've always loved and that just brings happiness every time you see it.

& As a Pairing

JADE and **CITRINE** are perfect companions for pyrite to enhance energies of prosperity and abundance. Use these crystals in any combination to improve financial or professional matters, and for all forms of abundance. **TIGER'S EYE** and pyrite also create a powerful pairing, blending the energies of the sun and earth to leave you strong and energized. Pyrite's iron-based cousin **HEMATITE** is another good match, as each stone enhances the grounding energies of the other.

JADE

CITRINE

HEMATITE

CITRINE

"THE MERCHANT'S STONE"

APPEARANCE

CITRINE is a form of quartz crystal characterized by its color, which can range from yellow to orange to light brown. Most citrine crystals are heat-treated amethyst. True citrine has more subtle coloration than the augmented bright orange/yellow versions.

MEANING

Often referred to as the "merchant's stone," citrine has long been associated with prosperity, abundance, and manifestation. Its sunny, enriching energy helps us to realize our potential in life.

RARITY

True, natural citrine is rare in nature, but heat-treated forms of other quartz crystals are widely available and these have similar properties.

FOR YOUR STAR SIGN

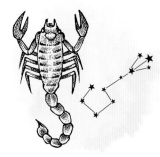

A birthstone for November (along with topaz), citrine connects with those who are born under the sign of Scorpio. Scorpios are passionate, dramatic, loving people, and full of life, making this golden gem a very fitting crystal companion. Citrine complements the best attributes of Scorpios—their ambition, drive, and tenacity—and softens the edges around their more difficult qualities of aggression and jealousy. A Scorpio personality combined with the golden ray of citrine makes for a truly unbeatable pairing.

IN A DAILY RITUAL

If you're seeking more prosperity and abundance in your life—and who isn't?—harness the energy of the "merchant stone" in this simple ritual. Carry a piece of citrine in your purse or wallet, or place a crystal in your office, studio, or workspace. This will invite the energy of abundance into your life.

In Reiki

Use citrine to help balance the solar plexus region, or anywhere your energy is feeling sluggish or imbalanced. This is a particularly handy crystal for body layouts and energy work because it does not have to be cleansed as often as other stones.

Angels & Deities

Citrine has a connection with the Greek goddess Demeter, who ruled over agriculture, harvest, and abundance.

WORKING WITH THE CHAKRAS

Sweet citrine is one of the preeminent stones for solar plexus chakra work. The solar plexus, called *manipura* in Sanskrit, is located just above the navel and is our center for personal power, self-esteem, and transformation. When our solar plexus chakra is out of balance, we may experience low self-confidence, have difficulty making decisions, or feel unmotivated or drained of energy. Wearing citrine on the body helps to balance and energize this chakra throughout the day, resulting in a more self-assured, successful, and radiant *you*.

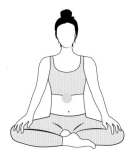

For Protection

Citrine is a supremely protective stone to keep on the body, or in your home or workspace. It transmutes negative energy to positive, surrounding us with a lightness at all times. Keeping citrine in the workplace, in particular, will help protect your business dealings and money matters.

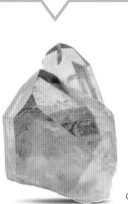

Citrine

IN A CRYSTAL GRID

Use the "Vesica Piscis" grid for this crystal (see page 122). Citrine is highly versatile in crystal grids and, like most forms of quartz, is compatible with a whole array of crystals. It will complement so many different grid themes, but the most natural choice is one to enhance abundance and prosperity. Try pairing with tiger's eye and peridot for a powerful, "abundant energy" grid. Use citrine in the focus stone position. Then use tiger's eye for the way stones and peridot for the desire stones. Each crystal's energy enhances that of the others exponentially. Place a personal item inside, such as coins or a business card, to hone your intention.

HEALING PROPERTIES

Mental & Emotional
Citrine has long held a connection to the sun, and like that life-giving celestial body, it imparts a warmth and rejuvenating energy. Citrine brings you into alignment with your self-will, potential, creativity, and personal power. Turn to citrine to increase motivation and activity, as well as to tackle fear and depression.

Spiritual
Citrine is a stone of light, on many different levels. It infuses the spirit with bright, positive energy and attracts us to the light in other people. This is why citrine is a stone of manifestation and abundance: the more we embody an energy of joy and positivity, the more we welcome that energy into our lives.

Physical
This sunny gemstone provides physical energy and has the power to invigorate the system. It supports the digestive system and healthy metabolic function. Use citrine if you suffer from any problems in the pancreas, spleen, or kidneys. Citrine can also be useful if you wish to maintain healthy skin.

& As a Pairing

Pair citrine with **TIGER'S EYE**, as its motivating energies enhance citrine's abundant energy, and with **CARNELIAN** for lower chakra energy. For abundance, pair citrine with **JADE** and **PERIDOT**. Citrine can also enhance the properties of **MOSS AGATE** and pairs well with other quartzes like **GOLDEN HEALER QUARTZ** and **CLEAR QUARTZ**. Both **TOPAZ** and **PYRITE** amplify citrine's energies of prosperity and joyfulness, while citrine can help manifest the lofty energies and inspiration of **AMETHYST**.

TIGER'S EYE

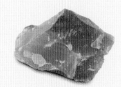

CARNELIAN

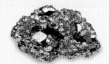

PYRITE

GOLDEN HEALER QUARTZ

"THE HEALER STONE"

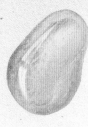

APPEARANCE

GOLDEN HEALER QUARTZ ranges in color from almost transparent yellow, to clear to darker opaque yellow, to opaque yellow/orange due to the presence of iron oxide. It is available in crystal points, carvings, tumbled stones, beads, and more.

MEANING

Golden healer quartz, as the name suggests, is a stone with deeply healing benefits, both for yourself and when working on others. It vibrates with the golden ray, tapping into the divine life-force energy.

RARITY

Golden healer is a moderately priced stone, as it is one of the rarer forms of quartz crystal and highly sought after in the metaphysical community.

IN A CRYSTAL GRID

Use the "Borrowmean Rings" grid for this crystal (see page 123). For health and healing use golden healer quartz as the focus stone. Add clear quartz points as way stones and selenite as desire stones, providing universal energy to heal yourself or another. Visualize the emotional or physical issue as you create and charge the grid, then envision this being healed—hold that thought in your mind's eye.

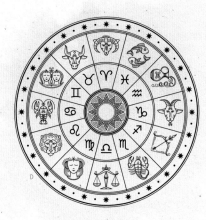

FOR YOUR STAR SIGN

Golden healer quartz is a crystal of the sun, and is unique in that it is equally suited to all astrological signs, amplifying the flow of healing energy through the body.

—— In Reiki ——

In Reiki or energy healing, nothing compares to the myriad uses for the golden healer quartz. Place this quartz anywhere there is an energy blockage in the body. An added benefit is that both sender and receiver receive the energetic benefits.

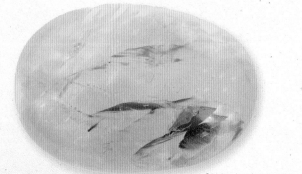

For Protection

When we speak of the golden ray of light, we are referring to a source of universal consciousness; some know it as Christ consciousness. It is a frequency that imparts divine wisdom and protection when called upon.

Golden healer quartz

IN A DAILY RITUAL

For this practice, place your golden healer quartz outside in bright sunlight for several hours to be cleansed and recharged. When you are ready, hold the stone over the top of your head. In your mind's eye, visualize golden light entering through the crown chakra. See this exquisite, golden light filling your body. Repeat as a mantra, silently or aloud: "I am light. There is no place where the universe ends and I begin."

Angels & Deities

Golden healer quartz is said to vibrate with the energy of Christ consciousness.

HEALING PROPERTIES

Mental & Emotional

The beauty of this sunny stone lies in its universal ability to heal damage and also to remove blockages. If you find yourself feeling stagnant, or struggling to "move on" in your life, call upon the golden healer. It carries within it the energy of the sun: powerful, renewing, and responsible for growth and abundance.

Spiritual

This stone is considered by many to be a "master healer" on so many levels. It raises our energetic frequency and allows us to receive divine messages and healing energy. Golden healer quartz also has the ability to connect us with spirit guides and to amplify intentions—making it a wonderful tool for manifestation.

Physical

Golden healer quartz makes a wonderful companion for anyone who is dealing with fatigue, sluggishness, or imbalances in any organ or physical system. This beautiful stone grants a reparative energy to the cells of the whole body.

WORKING WITH THE CHAKRAS

All the chakras benefit from the ability of golden healer quartz to repair blockages and reinstate a free flow of energy. The crown chakra in particular resonates strongly with the golden ray of light, as do the sacral and solar plexus chakras. Another unique quality is this stone's ability to align the higher and lower chakras. If you could choose only one crystal for all your chakra work, this golden gem would be an excellent candidate. Due to its iron content, it does emit an earthly, grounding energy.

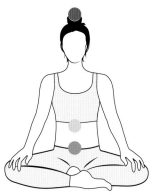

As a Pairing

Golden healer pairs beautifully with any member of the quartz crystal family, particularly its golden cousin, **CITRINE**. Combining with **SELENITE** will bring divine white light down into the body. Selenite also has the additional benefit of recharging the crystal, from which a golden healer can frequently benefit.

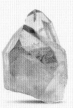

CITRINE

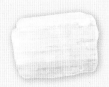

SELENITE

HONEY CALCITE

"THE STONE OF SWEET COMFORT"

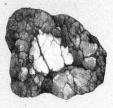

APPEARANCE

HONEY CALCITE, also known as golden or citrine calcite, is a very special variety of the massive calcite family of minerals. As its name suggests, it is light golden to amber or brown in color, and is mostly mined in Mexico.

MEANING

All forms of calcite have uplifting and purifying properties. However, you will find that honey calcite brings with it an added sense of self-assurance, psychic insight, and abundance.

RARITY

Calcite is one of the most abundant minerals on the planet. For this reason, honey calcite is quite affordable and attainable.

IN A DAILY RITUAL

One fun and effective way to infuse your space with healing crystal energy is by crystal-gridding your home. There's no better stone to choose for this than sweet honey calcite. Choose a few pieces in any form: raw, tumbled, towers, and so on, then place one piece in each corner of the home and one piece in the center of your home.

Angels & Deities

Native Americans considered calcite a holy stone, given to them by their gods and ancestors.

FOR YOUR STAR SIGN

Honey calcite is a perfect match for those born under Cancer, the sign of the crab. This astrological period welcomes the beginning of summer, resonating with calcite's warm, sunny energies. Cancerians are sensitive, loyal, and intuitive. But they can sometimes become unbalanced and overly emotional. Enter the golden form of calcite and its calming, balancing energy. At its core, honey calcite is a stone of comfort, which the Cancerian craves on a deep, spiritual level.

For Protection

Calcite is known to be very effective for its purifying energy. Honey calcite specifically attracts abundance and good fortune. It's great to wear on the body, keeping it in contact with the skin, or placed around the home or workspace.

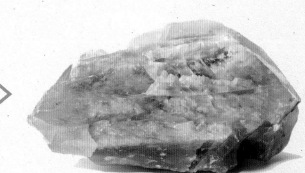

Honey calcite

WORKING WITH THE CHAKRAS

Honey calcite is special in terms of the number of chakras it works well with: the root, sacral, third eye, and crown chakras all make a connection. But its primary energy center is the solar plexus. This, our third chakra, is all about self-will, confidence, determination, and manifestation. Honey calcite makes the perfect match: filling us with an energy of self-sufficiency, strengthening our willpower, and reminding us that our capabilities are limitless. Honey calcite helps us to see ourselves in the truest, sunniest light. When we fully realize our own power, we can use it for the greatest good.

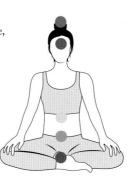

IN A CRYSTAL GRID

Use the "Metatron's Cube" grid for this crystal (see page 123). As a group, calcite makes up a significant portion of the earth's crust. Creating an all-calcite grid connects you with the beautiful energy of this stone, essentially linking you to the earth itself. Try a white or clear calcite as the focus stone surrounded with pink calcite as the way stones and honey calcite as the desire stones.

—— In Reiki ——

Honey calcite is an invaluable tool for Reiki healing sessions. It gently amplifies the energies of other crystals, imparts warmth and positivity during the session, and ensures that the sender remains free of unwanted energies during and after the healing.

HEALING PROPERTIES

Mental & Emotional

Honey calcite is empowering, yet it lifts you up in the gentlest of ways. It creates an important connection between the emotional and the intellectual mind, which can help to alleviate anxiety and insecurity. Turn to honey calcite if you feel in need of a little extra motivation, reassurance, or comfort.

Spiritual

Honey calcite constantly cleanses space, both physical and auric, and is an invaluable tool for meditation sessions. Its energies are sweet, strong, and purifying. Honey calcite does not provide us with all the answers; rather, it empowers us to realize that the spiritual insights and universal truths are already within our grasp.

Physical

Honey calcite brings balance to the glands and strengthens the immune system. It helps to dissolve calcification of the bones and balance overall calcium levels in the body. The bones and joints will benefit from working with this honey-hued gem, as will the pancreas, kidneys, and bladder.

& As a Pairing

Pair honey calcite with the rare **WULFENITE** to super-charge your lower chakras, enhance personal power, or strengthen the sex drive. In addition, try creating combinations with other colors of **CALCITE**—pink or green for extra heart-healing energy, or blue for meditative and spiritual pursuits. You'll find that the sunny energies of **AMBER** offer a perfect complement to the warm positivity of honey calcite.

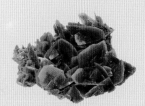

WULFENITE

CALCITE

AMBER

EMERALD

"THE STONE OF SUCCESSFUL LOVE"

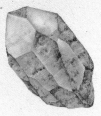

APPEARANCE

EMERALD is in the beryl family, along with its cousins blue aquamarine and pink morganite. A hexagonal crystal, emerald ranges in color from very dark to light, yellowish-green. The mineral can be either translucent or opaque.

MEANING

Due to its association with love, emerald is rumored to change color as a sign of infidelity in a relationship, and has been touted throughout history as a stone of prophecy and protection.

RARITY

Perfect specimens of emerald can be more valuable than those of diamond, although lower-quality mineral is easily acquired.

HEALING PROPERTIES

Mental & Emotional

Emerald is intensely healing for the heart, allowing us to bolster our self-love and love for others. It carries within its green ray of energy the rejuvenating power of spring, fresh growth, and new beginnings. This green gem also assists with mental clarity and memory.

Spiritual

Arising in ancient mysticism and lore, emerald has long held a prominent place in our collective human spirit. By balancing the emotions and heart center, it allows us to further our greater, spiritual journey. A stone of prophecy and transformation, emerald has been known for millennia as a bridge to the divine.

Physical

Use emerald to strengthen the heart and eyes, as well as to bolster the immune and nervous systems. The Greek philosopher Aristotle prescribed it to prevent epilepsy. Emerald assists in areas of mental clarity and memory, so is said to strengthen the brain. It can produce a detoxifying effect on the physical body as a whole.

For Protection

An ancient talisman for protection, emerald has often been worn by travelers embarking on long journeys, warriors as they go into battle, and anyone who is seeking to ward off an evil enchantment. Cleopatra was even said to gift emeralds to dignitaries to ensure their safe return home.

IN A DAILY RITUAL

Working with emerald when meditating can yield profound benefits within your day-to-day life. Use it to increase abundance in many different areas: love, wealth, or healing. Hold the crystal in your left hand and think to yourself or say aloud: "I open myself to divine love. I invite abundance to fill my life." Wearing emerald around the neck is a wonderful way to keep this affirmation present throughout the day.

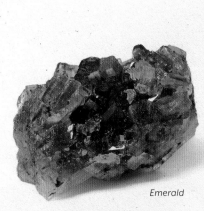

Emerald

FOR YOUR STAR SIGN

Emerald is connected to the planet Mercury, so working with this stone will strengthen that planetary influence in your horoscope. Mercury affects the areas of communication, intellect, and wisdom. It is the traditional birthstone for the month of May. The astrological signs Gemini, Virgo, and Taurus will derive particular benefit from working with this verdant gem. Someone requiring more Mercury energy in their life may find that they are struggling with anxiety, indecisiveness, or sluggishness. Wednesday is associated with Mercury, which makes it a good day to work with emerald to strengthen these attributes!

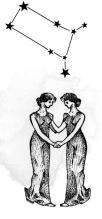

IN A CRYSTAL GRID

Use the "Tripod of Life" grid for this crystal (see page 123). Love is the greatest pursuit and meaning of life, but as vulnerable humans, we also want to keep our hearts safe from harm as much as possible. Tap into the ancient power of the "stone of successful love" in a grid designed to safely open the heart. Use rose quartz as the focus stone in the center of the grid. Place smoky quartz in the way stone position and finish with emerald as the desire stones. This recipe calls for love to enter our hearts and lives, while keeping us safe and protected from emotional harm.

———— In Reiki ————

In Reiki or crystal energy healing, position emerald over the heart for emotional healing—particularly if you want to remove emotional blockages in that area. You may also choose to place emerald on the third eye chakra to enhance areas of intuition or insight. Remember that emerald must be cleared often.

Angels & Deities

The energy of emerald calls upon the Archangel Raphael for divine protection and guidance. It has also been associated with the goddesses Venus and Aphrodite.

WORKING WITH THE CHAKRAS

Emerald is one of the most effective stones for working with the heart chakra. Like any muscle, the heart can grow sore and weary from time to time. Everyday matters of life and love take their toll on us, but we can turn to the rejuvenative energy of emerald for solace and healing. Anahata, the fourth chakra, located in the center of the chest, regulates our ability to love ourselves, our relationships with others, and our general emotional stability. Wearing a piece of emerald around this energy center can provide an intentional reminder throughout the day of the healing work that is being done.

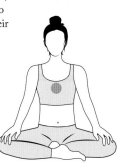

& As a Pairing

Pair emerald with **ROSE QUARTZ** to combine their heart-healing, love-filled energies, as they open the heart chakra. But if you are too emotionally vulnerable, pair with the grounding energy of **BLACK OBSIDIAN** or **SMOKY QUARTZ** for healthy boundaries and protection. Also pair emerald with other beryl minerals such as **MORGANITE** and **AQUAMARINE** since their energies vibrate at very compatible frequencies.

ROSE QUARTZ

BLACK OBSIDIAN

SMOKY QUARTZ

JADE

"THE STONE OF GOOD LUCK"

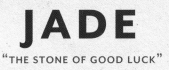

APPEARANCE

JADE is actually a term used to describe two different minerals: jadeite and nephrite. Although emerald green is the most commonly known form, it can be found in a rainbow of colors (we'll be focusing on the green variety here).

MEANING

Although Chinese culture is most often associated with this verdant stone, jade has been cherished in many different cultures across the globe for its appearance in ornamentation, strength in toolmaking, and association with good luck, harmony, and prosperity.

RARITY

Jadeite is the rarer and more valuable form, with deep green "imperial jade" from Myanmar being the rarest of all.

IN A DAILY RITUAL

Using jade in massage and beauty treatments has increased in popularity in recent years, although this practice has been popular in China for centuries. Use a special gua sha tool, facial roller, or simply a tumbled jade stone in order to reap the benefits of crystal massage work. The benefits include improved circulation and lymphatic drainage, and energetic detoxification.

FOR YOUR STAR SIGN

Jade connects with those ruled by the planet Venus, which governs love, beauty, and pleasure. This means individuals born under the signs of Taurus and Libra will have a special affinity for sweet jade. Driven, ambitious Taureans will make great use of jade's energy of prosperity and abundance. It also suits their penchant for the finer things in life. Librans fixate on balance and justice in all affairs, and jade will help keep the moral high ground in sight.

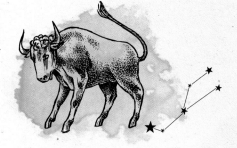

Angels & Deities

Chalchiuhtlicue is the Aztec goddess of bodies of water and fertility, and her name translates to "she who wears a jade skirt."

WORKING WITH THE CHAKRAS

Green jade connects deeply with the heart chakra. It is perhaps no coincidence that some of the most valuable gemstones—emerald, ruby, and jade—have been associated with this oh-so-sacred center of energy throughout history. Indeed, if anahata, the heart chakra, is unbalanced or blocked, nothing in life seems to work properly. Jade brings a singular steadiness to the heart and an energy that whispers: "It is all okay—always has been, always will be." Its use throughout human history is testament to the profound benefit of working with this verdant, heart-centered gem.

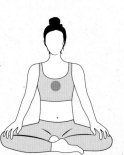

— In Reiki —

Jade wands are popular tools for energy healing with crystals. Using these or tumbled stones, try focusing around the chest and heart center. In general, jade is a supportive stone, so use on the body anywhere there is unease or imbalance.

For Protection

Jade talismans have been worn for thousands of years to bring protection and good luck. Similarly, jade carvings have been used in feng shui for protection and good energy in the home. Jade is believed to strengthen the chi (or life-force energy), thus warding off negative vibrations.

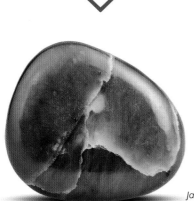

Jade

IN A CRYSTAL GRID

Use the "Vesica Piscis" grid for this crystal (see page 122). Choose jade stone to create a powerful grid for bringing wealth into your life. Remember that money is simply energy—working with crystals, energy healing, and financial transactions are all exchanges of energy. There is nothing unspiritual about seeking to better your financial situation. Combine the abundant energy of jade with citrine (also known as the "merchant's stone") and peridot for increased success, prosperity, and financial stability. Use citrine as the focus stone, peridot as the way stones, and jade as the desire stones. For a little extra oomph, place some coins inside the grid.

HEALING PROPERTIES

Mental & Emotional
The lush, green color of jade is no coincidence. It glows with the hue of growing things, and so imparts energies of growth, healing, and life-force energy. Jade calms anxiety and assists with mental health struggles. It bolsters self-confidence, helping us to acknowledge and ask for what we truly deserve.

Spiritual
Jade is a stone of abundance on every level. It helps us to identify our most highly esteemed qualities, those that we aspire to represent and then begin to manifest in our everyday life. Abundant love, compassion, generosity, forgiveness—these qualities flow more easily if you attune to the energy of jade.

Physical
It is said the name jade is derived from the Spanish *piedra de la ijada*, meaning "stone of the side," which may have been born out of its long-known effectiveness in treating problems of the kidneys, bladder, and spleen. It is generally detoxifying, and has been used for such purposes since ancient times.

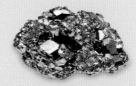

As a Pairing

In order to bring in abundance energy, pair jade with **PYRITE**, **CITRINE**, or **PERIDOT**. Jade emanates a gentle, heart-based energy, while the other crystals bring a more fiery vibration. Pair jade with other green- or pink-hued gems to enhance its heart chakra-opening energies.

PYRITE

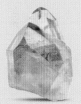

CITRINE

PERIDOT

MOLDAVITE

"THE EXTRATERRESTRIAL STONE"

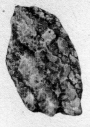

APPEARANCE

Moldavite is actually a tektite, a kind of natural glass formed by a meteoric impact almost 15 million years ago in what is now the Czech Republic. It is light to hunter green in color, and usually textured with what appear to be bubbles or swirls.

MEANING

Moldavite has a high frequency and so is not for beginners. This highly vibrational gem aids spiritual awakening and shields the aura from negative energy attacks. It's thought the Holy Grail was made of moldavite and that its otherworldliness may connect it to extraterrestrial energy.

RARITY

Authentic moldavite is quite valuable, and is increasing in value as many mines are being depleted.

WORKING WITH THE CHAKRAS

Moldavite is effective at unblocking all the chakras, but especially the heart and third eye energy centers. Unlike a softer companion such as rose quartz, moldavite works to blast through blockages of energy with an unrivaled intensity. Use it for deep emotional, heart-based healing work on the chest, or place on the brow, over the third eye, to tap into your intuition and reveal spiritual insights. Whatever your end goal is, moldavite will hasten your journey there. It is also very effective at stimulating *kundalini* energy, allowing us to access our deepest creative potential.

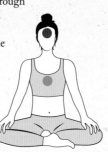

For Protection

Moldavite offers massive protection from negative energy and psychic attack by shielding the aura. It brings you into communication with your spirit guides—at which point you will notice synchronicities and "signs" in your day-to-day life—and they will bestow divine guidance and protection along your journey.

IN A DAILY RITUAL

Before working with moldavite, it is wise to cleanse the crystal to clear it of any unwanted energy. Natural spring water is a good method for cleansing this stone. Once your crystal is prepared, decide upon your intention. For healing/strengthening the heart and emotional body, place the moldavite on your chest and visualize gentle, green rays of light wrapping around you. Imagine all the love of the universe and cosmos: the endless, unfathomable sum of pure divine love. Imagine this entering your body, then repeat the mantra: "I am made of love, I am made of stars."

Angels & Deities

Moldavite holds a strong connection to Gaia, or Mother Earth, as well as extraterrestrial energies.

Moldavite

FOR YOUR STAR SIGN

All zodiac signs can benefit from the universally transformative powers of moldavite, a gift from the cosmos. Those born in spring, however, under the sign of Taurus, will have a particular connection with moldavite. Taureans may be rigid or stubborn, but nothing can shake up some old, worn-out patterns like the electrifying energy of moldavite. These individuals are also generally strong and stable enough to be able to withstand the intensity of this green gem.

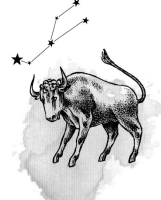

HEALING PROPERTIES

Mental & Emotional

Moldavite's intense energy can be transformative when healing old wounds and generational trauma. People sometimes find that working closely with moldavite brings them into repeated, difficult situations—personally, professionally, emotionally—the reason being that these are the trials we must go through in order to grow.

Spiritual

Nothing will accelerate your spiritual journey like meteoric moldavite. It will open you to divine guidance and help you realize your true path. Its energy cannot be overstated, so be prepared for a cosmic impact in your life as you work with it. Use in past-life regression and dreamwork, and to enhance telepathic abilities.

Physical

Just as moldavite can root out underlying emotional issues that may plague us, so too does it work to uncover the source of a physical ailment. It can have a rejuvenating effect on the body as a whole, reversing cellular damage and signs of aging. It has also been used as a talisman for women's health.

IN A CRYSTAL GRID

Use the "Metatron's Cube" grid for this crystal (see page 123). Since moldavite is a tektite and not a "crystal," its positioning in a crystal grid is flexible. However, due to its expense and energetic output, I suggest using a single piece as the focus stone. This would make a good grid to send loving-kindness to an individual or to humanity as a whole. Place herkimer diamonds in the way stone position and, lastly, use rose quartz as the desire stones. After completion, meditate on loving-kindness while feeling the grid's intense, heart-based, high-vibration energies radiate outward.

─── In Reiki ───

Moldavite can be an incredibly transformative crystal to use during Reiki healing sessions, but go slowly and make sure the receiver has some experience with this crystal beforehand. Place the stone above the head to stimulate the crown chakra for some very revelatory experiences! Be advised that working with moldavite often produces the "moldavite flush," a very palpable, warming sensation in the body that may be felt by both the sender and receiver.

& As a Pairing

Pair moldavite with **ROSE QUARTZ** to soften its intense vibrations. Use **TIGER'S EYE** as a companion for courage of the heart, when the lessons of moldavite feel too intense. Alternatively, to enhance the crown chakra connection and deepen its effects, pair it with **HERKIMER DIAMOND**.

ROSE QUARTZ

TIGER'S EYE

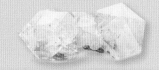

HERKIMER DIAMOND

MALACHITE

"THE STONE OF REJUVENATION"

APPEARANCE

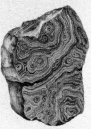

MALACHITE is an opaque, copper carbonate mineral, with bands of lighter to darker green. The swirling undulations of coloring are unlike any other stone: emblematic of its singular energetic presence. It is most often seen in cabochon or tumbled stone form.

MEANING

The word *malachite* is derived from the ancient Greek for "mallow" as it resembles the leaves of the mallow plant. This soft mineral has been ground and used as a pigment for millennia, including in Cleopatra's cosmetics.

RARITY

Malachite is an abundant mineral, making it easy to add to a crystal collection. Combined with other minerals, such as azurite or chrysocolla, it increases in rarity and price.

IN A DAILY RITUAL

Malachite can be a wonderful tool for finding areas of the body where we may unconsciously be holding tension or blocked energy. Doing a quick, daily "scan" of the body can be a lovely ritual. Simply glide a piece of malachite over your body, up and down the limbs, from the base of the spine to the top of the head, and observe any slight "snags." Spend some time throughout the day sending healing energy to those areas.

Angels & Deities

Malachite was associated with Hathor, the Egyptian goddess of love and fertility, as well as the goddesses Venus and Juno.

FOR YOUR STAR SIGN

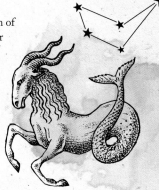

Individuals born under the sign of Capricorn will have a particular affinity with the lovely malachite. This captivating green stone helps to bring balance and optimism to the often serious and focused Capricorn. Capricorns may also find themselves struggling with self-imposed limitations, and malachite assists in removing those, as well as helping them to focus more on their positive qualities rather than any perceived areas of inadequacy.

For Protection

Malachite is one of the preeminent stones for protection, making it unusual for a stone of its coloring and mineralogical makeup. During the Middle Ages, it was used as protection from the evil eye and has been used to ward off negative spirits through the ages.

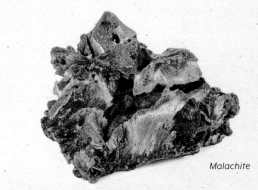

Malachite

WORKING WITH THE CHAKRAS

Although malachite is inarguably a heart chakra stone first and foremost, it is quite effective from the third eye chakra down to the solar plexus. It imparts various energies, from willpower and strength, to heart soothing, to psychic enhancement, making it a versatile and powerful tool for chakra energy work. It has a unique ability to release emotional blockages. You can begin to experiment with attuning yourself to the energy of this vibrant stone by placing it over your heart chakra in meditation, for short periods of time.

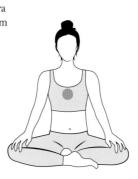

IN A CRYSTAL GRID

Use the "Spiral" grid for this crystal (see page 122). Malachite imparts a heart-based energy, making it ideal for grieving or healing. This is hard work, so ensure the aura is energetically shielded. Use a large smoky quartz as the focus stone, a heart chakra stone such as rose quartz or morganite as way stones, and malachite as desire stones. Charge the grid, imagining life-force energy keeping you safe and loved.

—— In Reiki ——

Due to its mineralogical makeup, malachite is a great tool for drawing out negative energy or disease from anywhere in the body. It is very energetically absorbent, but make sure to cleanse your malachite stone frequently—placing it outside to sit in moonlight or atop a selenite crystal are effective methods.

HEALING PROPERTIES

Mental & Emotional
Malachite imparts many of the heart-healing qualities of other green stones, but with a unique power and forcefulness. Make sure when you welcome malachite into your arsenal that you are ready for some real transformation. This lustrous mineral helps us to sever unhealthy emotional ties and invite forgiveness into our hearts.

Spiritual
Sometimes clearing the path for true spiritual growth is not an easy or pleasant process. Malachite can facilitate this and hold our hand for the ride. It reveals our largest obstacles and then gives solutions for dissolving them. It can also help us repair holes in our auric/energetic field and rid ourselves of karmic baggage.

Physical
Malachite is said to help reduce inflammation and provide a generally detoxifying effect on the body. It has long been associated with women's health, the regulation of menstrual cycles and for assisting in childbirth and early infant care.

& As a Pairing

For the enhancement of heart-based energies, nothing beats the combination of malachite and **MORGANITE**. The sweet vibration of morganite is a lovely match for malachite's intensity. Alternatively, to keep your heart and emotions safe and protected, try pairing malachite with **BLACK TOURMALINE** or **SMOKY QUARTZ**.

MORGANITE

BLACK TOURMALINE

SMOKY QUARTZ

CHRYSOPRASE

"THE STONE OF VENUS"

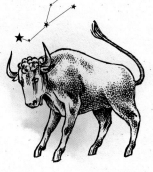

APPEARANCE
CHRYSOPRASE is a semitranslucent form of chalcedony, ranging in color from slightly yellow-green to deep green. It is one of the only green stones that gains its hue from nickel. Chrysoprase is usually available in cabochon and bead form.

MEANING
The name *chrysoprase* is derived from the Greek words for "golden" and "leek." It has held great value and significance across many cultures for millennia.

RARITY
Chrysoprase is one of the rarest forms of chalcedony, and yet it is relatively accessible and affordable. High-quality, faceted stones can fetch high prices.

FOR YOUR STAR SIGN
The month of May is traditionally associated with emerald, but chrysoprase makes an affordable alternative. The astrological signs Taurus and Gemini in particular may benefit from this relaxing, optimistic stone. For Taureans, chrysoprase was often carved into images of a bull in medieval times. Venus is the planet that rules chrysoprase, so anyone seeking to strengthen the Venus influence in their astrological chart may want to slip one of these gems into their pocket!

IN A DAILY RITUAL
Due to its connection with nature spirits and Mother Earth, this practice is ideal for an outside space—preferably conducted barefoot, so you can ground properly into the earth. Hold a piece of chrysoprase in your right hand and really try to soak in that green, verdant color/energy filling in any "crack" in your heart space. Use the following words as a mantra: "I am whole, I am joyous, I am free."

IN A CRYSTAL GRID
Use the "Seed of Life" grid for this crystal (see page 122). There's nothing more refreshing than some "spring cleaning" and it doesn't have to take place in spring! Clearing out, sprucing up, and revitalizing an area—whether a living, work, or outside space—can bring fresh energy to your outlook and daily actions. After you've decluttered, remodeled, or cleaned out a space, set up this grid to finish the work of inviting new energy in and clearing stagnant energy out. Use clear quartz as the focus stone and add chrysoprase as way stones and amethyst as desire stones.

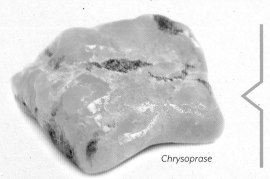

Chrysoprase

For Protection
Chrysoprase is believed to offer protection from negative entities, energy, and even dreams. According to legend, it was a favorite gemstone of Alexander the Great, who wore it into battle, believing it would keep him safe from harm. As the story goes, after one successful conquest, he left the gemstone on the riverbank while bathing. A serpent made off with the green gem, and Alexander never won another campaign.

Angels & Deities

Chrysoprase was once referred to as the "stone of Venus," and can also be used to connect to Mother Earth and nature spirits.

———— In Reiki ————

Chrysoprase is an excellent healing tool for chakra work as it has a very balancing energy and effect. It can be very effective in creating a connection or energetic link between the solar plexus and heart chakras during a Reiki session.

HEALING PROPERTIES

Mental & Emotional
Chrysoprase may assist you with achieving emotional equilibrium. Its special connection with the natural world lends the wearer/user a feeling of everything being in perfect, divine order. It imparts a joyous and optimistic energy, and can be useful at times when you are feeling mentally overwhelmed.

Spiritual
Through its heart-based energy and connection to the natural world, chrysoprase offers a doorway to deep, spiritual insights. This luminous gem teaches us that no matter what the question, love is always the answer. This realization and acceptance brings connection, prosperity, and compassion into our day-to-day lives.

Physical
Similar to its detoxifying effect on the emotions, chrysoprase can support the physical body to cleanse and rejuvenate itself. It is particularly effective in strengthening the heart, eyes, liver, and kidneys. Chrysoprase also helps to support our largest organ, the skin, and can impart a more youthful appearance overall.

WORKING WITH THE CHAKRAS

Like most green stones, chrysoprase connects very strongly with the heart chakra, also known as anahata. In fact, the energy of chrysoprase brings to mind the translation of the ancient Sanskrit term *anahata*, which means "unhurt, unbeaten, unstruck," as it helps us to overcome childhood trauma and even generational trauma from previous lifetimes. Releasing ourselves from this burden allows us to operate in an openhearted way—not that we move forward with naïveté, but are simply freed of the jaded and bitter energy that can result from disappointment and heartbreak.

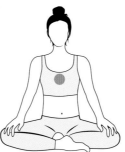

& As a Pairing

My personal favorite pairing for chrysoprase is **AMETHYST**—the energies complement each other so beautifully. Chrysoprase connects our heart to the earthly realm, while amethyst gently invokes a higher, spiritual vibration. Venturing further in that direction, pairing chrysoprase with **DANBURITE** or **PHENACITE** is a wise choice, as this provides an earthly tether for deep, spiritual work.

AMETHYST

DANBURITE

PHENACITE

MOSS AGATE

"THE STONE OF THE EARTH"

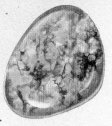

APPEARANCE

MOSS AGATE is technically a form of chalcedony, with inclusions of green, "mossy," dendritic mineral. The stone can be clear or somewhat opaque, and is usually found in tumbled or cabochon form.

MEANING

Moss agate is associated with abundance and wealth. It symbolizes luck, healing, and growth, and a connection with Mother Earth. Farmers in the past would scatter the stone across their land to ensure a bountiful harvest.

RARITY

Moss agate is a semiprecious stone, and a relatively accessible and affordable crystal to add to a collection.

HEALING PROPERTIES

Mental & Emotional

This stone provides a great feeling of emotional balance. It is particularly useful when your emotions feel erratic, overly intense, or traumatic. It seems to impart the sense of tranquility you feel after spending time in nature. It is also said to resolve imbalances between the left and right sides of the brain.

Spiritual

When embarking on any spiritual work or journey, you need to stay grounded. Moss agate provides that stability, due to its strong connection to the earth. When we feel safe and supported, the spirit can discover new depths of divine wisdom. It can also help sever karmic attachments from the past or even past lives.

Physical

Moss agate strengthens the immune system, and provides a balancing, stabilizing effect on all systems of the body. It is a particular friend to midwives and mothers, providing a strong, calming energy during childbirth.

IN A DAILY RITUAL

Use moss agate to call upon spirits of nature for rejuvenation, personal growth, or a deeper connection to the earth itself. Find a spot outside in nature that feels peaceful and inviting. This could be a beach, stream, bit of forest, or simply your own backyard. Sit down and close your eyes, holding a piece of moss agate in your right hand. Begin to visualize tendrils of energy swirling in the earth beneath you. Invite this healing energy to enter your feet, move up your legs, into your torso, and up through the crown of your head. Feel yourself connecting to the earth, the air, the light. Then say aloud or silently to yourself: "I am open to the wisdom and energy of the earth."

FOR YOUR STAR SIGN

Those born under the sign of Virgo will find a fitting companion in moss agate. Virgoans can often be detail-oriented and overly critical, and can benefit from the grounding energy of this crystal, which reminds us all to keep everything in perspective and let go of small trivialities. Moss agate encourages us to follow our intuition and heart-centered decision-making, which can be very useful practices for a Virgo.

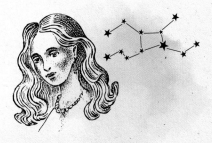

WORKING WITH THE CHAKRAS

As a green crystal, moss agate claims a strong heart chakra connection. It emits a lower energetic vibration than other crystals, and so provides a gentle space for difficult, heart-based healing work. Also, due to its grounding and stabilizing energy, it can be effective when working with the root chakra. Remember that the root chakra must be clear and allow the free flow of energy for any of the higher chakras to function optimally. Due to moss agate's unique ability to clear energetic blockages, it can be used in conjunction with other stones to clear and restore balance to any chakra.

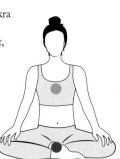

For Protection

Moss agate offers gentle protection around the aura—or energy field—that encompasses the body. Ancient warriors, shamans, and priests have all called upon the fortifying, protective qualities of this special stone. It is a perfect choice to wear as a necklace, ideally at heart-length, to harness its soothing vibrations through the day.

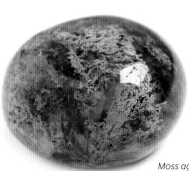

Moss agate

Angels & Deities

Archangel Raphael, the angel of healing, is connected to the energy of moss agate. You can also use this crystal to call upon Gaia, or Mother Earth, herself.

—— In Reiki ——

Moss agate is singularly beneficial in Reiki because it has the ability to reopen blocked pathways of energy throughout the body. Place a piece of moss agate on the body wherever you feel there is a blockage, or restriction, of energy.

IN A CRYSTAL GRID

Use the "Flower of Life" grid for this crystal (see page 122). Choose moss agate to create a grid to honor Mother Earth, nature spirits, or the changing of the seasons. This is a lovely ritual for the spring equinox and summer solstice. Use citrine as the focus stone, symbolic of the sun at the center of our solar system. Surround with clear quartz points as way stones, directing energy outward toward moss agate as the desire stones. Embellish with natural elements like flower petals, mushrooms, moss, or acorns.

& As a Pairing

Like a plant growing upward toward the light, moss agate seeks out the sunny energies of **CITRINE**, **PERIDOT**, and **AMBER**. Citrine and peridot radiate warmth and life-giving energy, allowing the properties of moss agate to bloom fully. Amber brings in an extra element of earth energy, enhancing the grounding effects of moss agate.

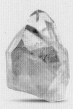

CITRINE

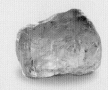

PERIDOT

AMBER

PERIDOT

"THE STONE OF PROSPERITY"

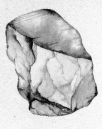

APPEARANCE
Peridot ranges from a yellow color to dark green, but is usually seen with a light- or olive-green tone. It is also known as olivine, and derives its coloration from the presence of iron.

MEANING
The energy of the sun seems to infuse this verdant stone. Since ancient times, it has been thought to provide rejuvenation, prosperity, abundance, and protection.

RARITY
Peridot is an abundant and affordable crystal, although gem-quality specimens are extremely rare. Such is its beauty, peridot is sometimes confused with emerald.

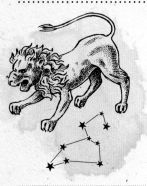

FOR YOUR STAR SIGN
Peridot is the official birthstone for August. It is associated with the sign of Leo, which is not surprising given that this lion's sign is ruled by the sun. Peridot has had a connection with the energy of the sun since ancient times—it is even said that the ancient Egyptians referred to it as "the gem of the sun." Leo is also said to govern the heart and solar plexus chakras, providing another strong connection to this green gem.

Angels & Deities
In Hawaiian legend, peridot is said to be the tears of the goddess Pele. It also carries a connection to the fairy realm and nature spirits.

——— In Reiki ———
Place peridot over the solar plexus region for the relief of tension and anxiety. Position over the heart for a boost in "light-hearted" energy, to increase vitality, or to allow for feelings of forgiveness. When the peridot is in its ideal placement for healing, you may feel a palpable warmth radiating through the body.

IN A DAILY RITUAL
Peridot is a perfect tool for any prosperity ritual. Prosperity and abundance, of course, are not limited to matters of money, but also encompass areas of love, health, and security. Identify in which way you wish your life to flourish, and sit comfortably with a peridot stone in your left hand. Visualize what you desire, and meditate on the words: "I welcome abundance into my life."

For Protection
Peridot was worn by the ancient Romans and Greeks as a talisman to ward off enchantment and evil spirits. It is suggested that Cleopatra wore it for this very reason. It is said to send any negative energies back to their source.

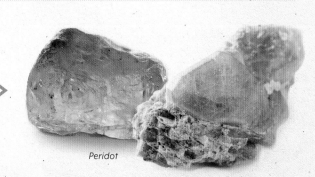

Peridot

HEALING PROPERTIES

Mental & Emotional
Do you frequently find yourself feeling sluggish, anxious, or unable to focus on the positives in life? If so, find solace in peridot. It can increase mental clarity, help to overcome negative thought patterns, and introduce the concept of abundance to our lives—in all its forms.

Spiritual
When we open ourselves to the limitless possibilities of the universe, the spirit blossoms as a flower in midsummer sunlight. We connect to a universal source of light, love, compassion, and growth. Clairvoyant abilities may be heightened, and you can attune to true abundance in many different guises.

Physical
The curative properties of peridot are nothing new, as ancient medicinal goblets were encrusted with this golden gem. It has long been thought to have a detoxifying effect on the body, which is helpful for liver function and also issues with metabolism and digestion. Peridot is also associated with anti-aging benefits.

IN A CRYSTAL GRID
Use the "Seed of Life" grid for this crystal (see page 122). Choose peridot to create a grid to increase abundance, especially in nonmaterial form (that is, in love, health, friendship). Use citrine as the focus stone and surround with peridot as the way stones and jade as the desire stones. Accent with rose or clear quartz pieces. If you can, add red clover flowers or cinnamon, as these are known to increase prosperity and abundance, and certainly add a touch of sweetness. Spend time visualizing all the wonderful things you are inviting into your life—and watch them manifest.

WORKING WITH THE CHAKRAS
Peridot creates an energetic connection between the solar plexus and heart chakras. An unbalanced solar plexus chakra, or *manipura* in Sanskrit, will manifest in poor self-esteem, lack of motivation, and weak willpower. In turn, this will eventually affect the heart center, as all the chakras are interconnected. Periodot delivers a one-two punch to realign this highway of energy. Strengthening the solar plexus, and our deepest sense of self, the heart gradually blossoms as we begin to attract the love we deserve. Wearing a long necklace of peridot is an effective way to bring attention to these energy centers.

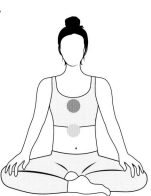

As a Pairing

MOSS AGATE pairs well with this sunny gem—the energies of light (peridot) and growth (moss agate) make a beautiful synergy. To amplify the inherent energies of peridot, use it with **CITRINE** or **JADE** as they share an ability to invite prosperity and generosity into your life, and one increases the energetic output of the other. Conversely, you can use peridot to amplify the sunny, radiant energies of **AMBER**—their combined energies are helpful for sacral and solar plexus chakra work and for depression.

MOSS AGATE

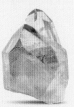

CITRINE

JADE

LAPIS LAZULI

"THE STONE OF WISDOM"

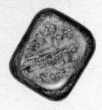

APPEARANCE

LAPIS LAZULI is composed of a combination of minerals, mainly lazurite (from which it derives its signature deep blue coloration), calcite, and flecks of pyrite. It can look solid blue to mottled, with the pyrite giving a subtle glimmer.

MEANING

Since ancient times, lapis lazuli has been associated with royalty, wisdom, intellect, and spirituality. The word *lapis* is derived from the Latin for "stone" and *lazuli* from the Persian *lazhward*, which means "blue."

RARITY

Although once considered more valuable than gold, lapis lazuli is quite affordable these days—however, good-quality specimens can still fetch high prices.

HEALING PROPERTIES

Mental & Emotional

Lapis lazuli calms an overly anxious mind, promoting peacefulness and clear thinking. It encourages self-awareness and the ability to see ourselves and our issues as parts of a greater whole. It is known as a stone of truth and can be relied upon to impart honesty, communication, and insight.

Spiritual

Lapis lazuli raises our awareness and connects us to a wellspring of divine wisdom. It has been used as a pigment through the ages, most notably by Michelangelo in the Sistine Chapel, and connects to a sacred source of inspiration. Use lapis lazuli to tap into your inherent psychic ability and increase your powers of intuition.

Physical

Turn to lapis lazuli for any issues you may have around the throat, larynx, vocal cords, or thyroid. This beautiful stone has proved helpful when dealing with hearing problems and chronic migraines. You can also use lapis lazuli to soothe a frazzled nervous system or strengthen a lagging immune system.

For Protection

Lapis lazuli has been associated with the cosmos and heavenly energy for as long as humans have mined it from the earth, making it the perfect talisman for protection. It is said to have the power to dispel negativity from life and to enhance our powers of intuition, thus empowering us to better safeguard our own energy.

IN A DAILY RITUAL

The ancient Egyptians believed this deep blue stone was connected to the night sky and the higher realms beyond. Try meditating outside at night, beneath starlight, with a piece of lapis lazuli in your hand or held up to the third eye chakra. Imagine the ancient stone is connecting you to the cosmos, the heavens, the spirit realm…

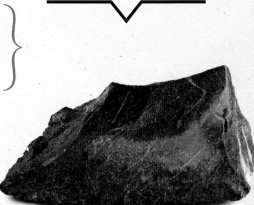

Lapis lazuli

IN A CRYSTAL GRID

Use the "Tripod of Life" grid for this crystal (see page 123), calling on lapis lazuli to enhance your intuition. Work on opening the third eye chakra and grow your psychic ability by tapping into the energy of this timeless stone. Place pieces of lapis lazuli in the desire stone position and combine with turquoise in the way stone position and amethyst as the focus stone. Spend a few minutes each day meditating with this grid for a week and observe changes in your intuitive ability as well as day-to-day synchronicities.

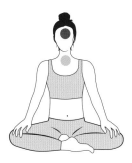

WORKING WITH THE CHAKRAS

Lapis lazuli corresponds with two chakras: the throat and the third eye. Its reputation as a stone of truth and expression aligns it perfectly with vishuddha, the throat chakra. When this chakra is balanced, we can express our truth and needs, and receive communication from others in an open and productive way. Moving up the body, we reach the third eye chakra (or ajna), which governs our intuition, psychic ability, and connection to the spirit world. Lapis lazuli works wonderfully with this chakra, in keeping with its ancient reputation as a bridge between the realms.

—— In Reiki ——

Lapis lazuli is an effective stone in Reiki healing for activating or balancing the throat and third eye chakras. It is also helpful for the sender to meditate with lapis lazuli before a treatment, to intuit where healing may be needed.

Angels & Deities

One of the oldest deities associated with lapis lazuli is the Sumerian goddess Inanna, who represented love and the underworld.

FOR YOUR STAR SIGN

While lapis lazuli is claimed as an alternative birthstone for both September and December, it is Sagittarius that has a special bond with this blue stone. The sign of the archer is adventurous, curious, and always seeking to propel herself forward in life. Lapis lazuli helps to calm this sign's sometimes erratic gusts of energy, so keeping Sagittarians on an even keel. Similarly, Sagittarius can get carried away and speak without thinking— lapis lazuli's link with the throat chakra can help in this area.

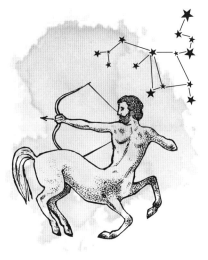

& As a Pairing

BLACK ONYX makes a powerful pairing with lapis lazuli, being highly protective and blocking negative energies—helpful when on a spiritual path paved by this blue stone. Pair lapis with **TURQUOISE** or **BLUE LACE AGATE**, to strengthen the throat chakra, and with **FLUORITE** to enhance intellectual ability and improve mental clarity. Gain an unparalleled intellectual boost by pairing lapis lazuli with **SAPPHIRE**.

BLACK ONYX

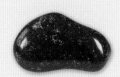

TURQUOISE

BLUE LACE AGATE

SAPPHIRE

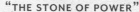

"THE STONE OF POWER"

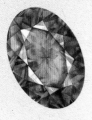

APPEARANCE

SAPPHIRE is the gem form of the mineral corundum, most commonly blue in color. Red corundum is known as ruby and any other color, including clear, yellow, orange, green, purple, pink, brown, or black, is categorized as sapphire.

MEANING

Sapphire has long been associated with royalty, nobility, power, romance, and faith. For millennia, the blue sapphire has represented the cosmos and our connection with divinity and higher wisdom.

RARITY

One of the four precious gemstones—the others being diamond, ruby, and emerald—a high-quality sapphire is quite rare and costly.

FOR YOUR STAR SIGN

Sapphire is the traditional Western birthstone for the month of September. However, its zodiacal association is a subject of much debate. It has been linked with Taurus, Gemini, Virgo, Libra, Capricorn, and Aquarius. What is agreed upon is the gem's relationship with the planet Saturn. Since Capricorn is ruled over by that dominant planet, the pairing of sapphire and the sign of the sea-goat makes sense. Methodical, driven Capricorn is perfectly matched by the energy of powerful, intellect-driven sapphire.

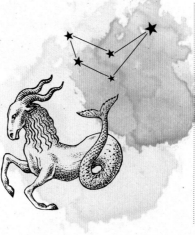

IN A DAILY RITUAL

Use sapphire in an easy, everyday meditation to open and strengthen the third eye chakra and your inherent psychic abilities. Find a comfortable seat and sit with a straight back and relaxed shoulders, neck, jaw, and face. Holding a piece of sapphire in your nondominant hand, lift the stone to touch just between the eyes. Imagine a brilliant indigo-blue light radiating outward from this spot.

—— In Reiki ——

Use sapphire on the body for healing work around the neck and throat, or on the forehead between the brows—in the third eye area.

Angels & Deities

Sapphire is associated with Apollo, the Greek and Roman god of the sun and prophecy.

WORKING WITH THE CHAKRAS

Different-colored sapphires correspond to various chakras, but for this section we'll focus on the most famous, the blue sapphire gem. This precious stone is unique in that it connects with both the third eye and the throat chakras. The third eye chakra governs our sense of intuition and ability to connect with higher consciousness. The throat chakra controls our ability to speak our truth, communicate clearly with others, and advocate for ourselves. When these two centers are both balanced and allow a free flow of energy, you are truly standing in your own power—with sapphire as your guide.

For Protection

*Sapphire takes its place among
the ranks of ancient talismans for
protection. It was said to repel sorcery,
redirect spells back to their sender,
banish evil spirits, and protect against
poisonous creatures. The famous
traveler Sir Richard Frances Burton
took a sapphire with him wherever he
went for protection and good luck.*

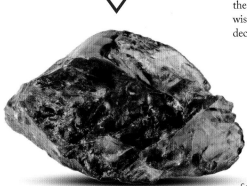

Sapphire

IN A CRYSTAL GRID

Use the "Metatron's Cube" grid for
this crystal (see page 123). For crystal
gridding and other rituals, you need not
worry about gem-quality specimens;
rough/raw stones are readily available
and very effective. Harness the ancient
wisdom of sapphire when you find
yourself at a crossroads in life, in times
of transition, or if there is a big decision
to be made. Place a large piece of clear
quartz in the center of the grid as the
focus stone. Place sapphire in the desire
stone position, combining with lapis
lazuli in the way stone position—for
the ultimate combination of ancient
wisdom, intuitive energy, and blessed
decision-making.

HEALING PROPERTIES

Mental & Emotional
Sapphire has always been linked to wisdom and the intellect. It
does not seem coincidental that this gem has traditionally adorned
rulers and those in positions of power; it brings a bold strength
and decisiveness. Emotionally, it allows us to break free of negative
patterns, ridding ourselves of heavy energy and self-doubt.

Spiritual
For millennia, the sapphire has been associated with the heavens
and our connection to the divine. It was worn by the ancient Greeks
when meeting the Oracle at Delphi, highly prized by early Buddhists,
and mentioned several times in the Bible. It may help with astral
journeying, past-life work, and dream recall.

Physical
The energy of the sapphire in physical healing is that of balance. It is
said to help those who are suffering from thyroid issues, migraines/
headaches, or vertigo. The mineral used to be ground into powder
and ingested to treat problems with eyesight and symptoms such as
fever and mouth ulcers.

As a Pairing

Pair sapphire with the only
other blue gem so rich in history
and reverence, **LAPIS LAZULI**,
for an unparalleled boost to
the intellect and higher mind.
Additionally, for a balance of
different energies, combine with
its corundum cousin, **RUBY**.
This play of heavenly and fiery
energies is effective in bringing
all chakras into alignment.

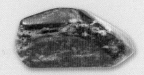

LAPIS LAZULI

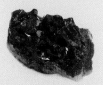

RUBY

AQUAMARINE

"THE MERMAID'S STONE"

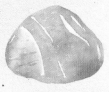

APPEARANCE

AQUAMARINE is the light blue variety of the mineral beryl—a family whose cousins include morganite and emerald. Crystals can form as perfect hexagonal shapes and have a hard, glassy appearance, ranging from a pale to deep blue color.

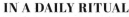

MEANING

Much like its namesake, the sea, aquamarine has a purifying and tranquilizing effect on our energy field. It has been used for millennia as a symbol of protection and was historically dubbed the "mermaid's stone."

RARITY

Although aquamarine is readily available, the more intensely colored specimens are on the rare and more valuable side.

WORKING WITH THE CHAKRAS

As with most blue-hued stones, aquamarine works strongly with the throat chakra. This is our fifth chakra, known in Sanskrit as *vishuddha*, which translates to "especially pure." Maintaining a healthy and balanced throat chakra allows us to access our deep inner truth—and to share that authentic state of being with the world. It enhances our creativity and ability to communicate. Aquamarine also speaks to the heart chakra, anahata, and creates an important connection between these two energy centers.

IN A DAILY RITUAL

Aquamarine is a perfect tool to use during any meditation, although one of the most enjoyable uses may be for a bathtime ritual—to harness the full, mermaid energy of this stone.

– Draw your bath mindfully.
– Set an intention to slow down and recharge from your day.
– Add calming essential oils—lavender, rose, or chamomile.
– Hold the stone between your throat and heart as you focus on its restorative energy.

—— In Reiki ——

Use the stone where there is heat, irritation, or tension in the body. For an overall cleansing and calming effect, place aquamarine over closed eyelids or the throat, or between the throat and the heart.

For Protection

In ancient times, aquamarine was used by sailors as a talisman of protection and good fortune, and its power in that area still remains strong. For those who travel often or live by the water, this is the crystal for you. Keep a stone in your pocket or luggage, or around your neck.

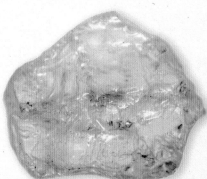

Aquamarine

IN A CRYSTAL GRID

Use the "Tripod of Life" grid for this crystal (see page 123). Aquamarine, emerald, and morganite are all forms of beryl, so share a similar energetic vibration and create a potent, uplifting, and visually stunning grid. The position of the stones is interchangeable depending on the intention, but to invite more positivity and joy, use morganite as the focus stone, aquamarine as the way stones, and emerald as the desire stones.

Angels & Deities

Aquamarine creates a spiritual connection with the guardian angels Vehuiah and Haaiah. It is associated with the Chinese goddess Guan Yin, deity of mercy and unconditional love, and patron saint of sailors.

&

As a Pairing

Aquamarine, **MORGANITE**, and **EMERALD** are all forms of the mineral family beryl—a silicate mineral found all over the world. As a result, they make a beautiful symphony when they are combined, vibrating beautifully together and each enhancing the unique qualities of the others. As a water element stone, aquamarine also loves the company of **LARIMAR** and **PEARL**.

HEALING PROPERTIES

Mental & Emotional
Aquamarine invites peace of mind and mental clarity due to its cooling and soothing effect on hotheaded behavior and thinking. A stone for the throat chakra, it invites us to discover our deepest inner truths and to assimilate that self-knowledge and intuition into our everyday lives.

Spiritual
An intensely detoxifying stone, aquamarine allows us to rid ourselves of toxic and destructive thinking, behavior, and energy. Its ancient association with the ocean imbues us with a steady serenity and allows us to access our highest selves, tapping into our telepathic and clairvoyant abilities.

Physical
Aquamarine is a stone of the breath and the throat. It is helpful for soothing chronic allergies and respiratory illnesses. Aquamarine can also be useful for regulating the hormones and to deal with vision problems that are caused by "tired eyes."

FOR YOUR STAR SIGN

The birthstone for March, aquamarine is most often associated with the zodiac sign of Pisces, the last sign of the astrological year. Pisceans make a perfect pairing with this aquatic gem. However, the surrounding signs of Aquarius and Aries may also find deep crystal companionship with aquamarine as well. While the constellation of Pisces looms in the sky, we find ourselves awash with reflection, fluidity of emotion, and creativity—all trademark gifts of this special stone.

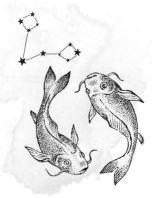

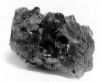

MORGANITE

EMERALD

LARIMAR

PEARL

TURQUOISE

"THE STONE OF LIFE"

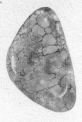

APPEARANCE

TURQUOISE is an opaque, copper-based mineral found in shades of blue, green, or yellow, with an evenly toned, medium blue being the most sought after. It usually displays a distinctive webbing called matrix, which is a glimpse of the host rock in which it formed.

MEANING

The word *turquoise* is derived from the old French word for "Turkish" due to the trade routes in this area. It was considered sacred by ancient civilizations like the Egyptians, Chinese, Persians, Aztecs, and Native Americans.

RARITY

Watch out for fake or dyed "turquoise." True turquoise is fairly easy to obtain and yet it ranges in value, with top-quality pieces fetching high prices.

IN A CRYSTAL GRID

Use the "Seed of Life" grid for this crystal (see page 122). Ancient Tibetans called turquoise the "sky stone," as it was thought to be a gift from the heavens. Honor turquoise's sacred past and spiritual power with clear quartz as the focus stone, turquoise as the way stones, and Tibetan quartz as the desire stones.

IN A DAILY RITUAL

With its connection to the neck and the throat chakra, an effective way to work with turquoise on a daily basis is by wearing it as a necklace. This is especially helpful when you're speaking in public, working in a group of people, or attempting a creative project of some sort.

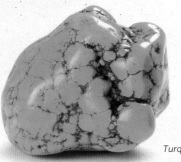

Turquoise

For Protection

Turquoise has always been seen as a stone of protection and good fortune, particularly if, according to legend, it is given by a friend. In ancient times, turquoise amulets were worn by soldiers and horses going into battle. It is said to change color to warn of infidelity, danger, or health problems.

FOR YOUR STAR SIGN

Turquoise is a birthstone for the month of December, and connects with the astrological sign of Sagittarius. The theme of the turquoise stone is bridging the gap between worlds, and the very image of Sagittarius represents that beautifully: the archer pulling back his bow. Jupiter is the ruling planet, the Roman god of the turquoise-blue sky. Turquoise amplifies Sagittarius's inherent intuitive abilities and provides the confidence to share that innate wisdom with the world.

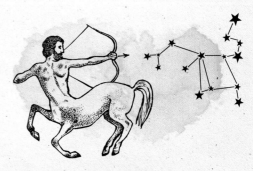

HEALING PROPERTIES

Mental & Emotional
Turquoise was said to unite the earth and the sky, male and female energies, yin and yang, providing an overall sense of balance and wholeness. It can be used to bring a state of calmness to the mind and emotions, which is helpful for anyone suffering from anxiety or depressive disorders.

Spiritual
Having the ability to unite the heavens and earth means turquoise can help us to align with our true spiritual purpose in life. Turquoise carries an element of purification, which assists in clearing away any toxicity or energetic debris around us. We can step into our true power and inner wisdom with the aid of turquoise.

Physical
Turquoise can be helpful for alleviating ear, nose, or throat problems. It can also be used to balance any systems within the body that are impaired and to support the absorption of nutrients. Turquoise increases energy levels and can be useful for combating fatigue or a feeling of sluggishness.

—— In Reiki ——
Use turquoise in the greener tones for heart-opening work and bluer specimens around the neck and throat. These also make a strong connection between the throat and third eye chakras.

Angels & Deities
Turquoise was linked to the Egyptian sky goddess Hathor, along with countless Native American deities.

WORKING WITH THE CHAKRAS
Turquoise is mainly associated with the area of vishuddha, the throat chakra, which governs communication: the way we receive and convey information, the way we speak to ourselves, the way we honor our own inner truth. It is said to bridge the inner and outer worlds, thus utilizing turquoise's ability to bring two worlds together. This center is also linked to our inner creativity and outward expression of that. The Sanskrit term *vishuddha* means "especially pure" since this energy center connects to the purification of the body, mind, and spirit.

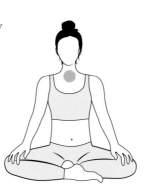

As a Pairing
Combine turquoise with **LARIMAR** for an unbeatable cocktail of relaxing, soothing energies. **LAPIS LAZULI** intensifies turquoise's connection to spirit and intuition. Turquoise has always been revered in Tibet, so combine with **TIBETAN QUARTZ** to access that spiritual energy.

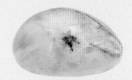

LARIMAR

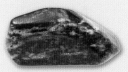

LAPIS LAZULI

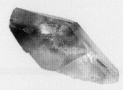

TIBETAN QUARTZ

LABRADORITE

"THE STONE OF MAGIC"

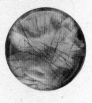

APPEARANCE

LABRADORITE is a variety of feldspar, discovered in rocks in Labrador. In Inuit legend, the northern lights were frozen in the rocks and found by a warrior who tried to free them with his spear. Some of the lights remained, creating labradorite's mystical shimmer.

MEANING

Labradorite is synonymous with mysticism, magic, and transformation. One look at this glimmering stone is enough to affirm that it carries some otherworldly energy and powers.

RARITY

Some colors of labradorite are rarer than others, but in general this is a relatively abundant crystal. It is usually found in tumbled or cabochon form.

IN A DAILY RITUAL

Use labradorite in a daily practice to increase telepathy and tap into your intuitive abilities. Hold the stone in your left hand, close your eyes, and focus on opening the mind's eye—just like opening a tiny door. Imagine benevolent messages/ messengers from the universe stepping through the doorway. Remain alert and open throughout the day for signs and displays of synchronicity.

FOR YOUR STAR SIGN

Mystical labradorite is particularly beneficial for those born under the sign of Pisces. Naturally intuitive and imaginative, Pisceans respond well to this flashy crystal friend. The season of Pisces represents a natural time of change, transition, and transformation for everyone. Labradorite is, above all else, a touchstone for transformation. It can support you during periods of growth, which this season of the zodiac calendar tends to foster.

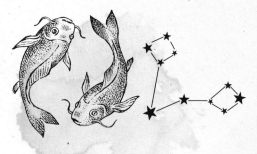

Angels & Deities

Labradorite has a connection with Arianrhod, the Welsh goddess of the moon, stars, and the northern lights.

WORKING WITH THE CHAKRAS

Its ability to connect to spiritual realms makes labradorite a perfect stone for working with the third eye chakra. When this chakra is blocked, you may find yourself feeling unmotivated, stagnant, or disconnected in your life. If the third eye is overactive, you may feel overwhelmed or exhausted from sensory overload. An open and balanced third eye is the goal, which labradorite seeks to create. This state creates a sense of mental and emotional clarity, optimism, and openness to intuition. You feel open to receiving messages from the universe, and able to assimilate those into your life.

In Reiki

Although labradorite is primarily a third eye crystal, it may be used in energy healing anywhere from the solar plexus to the crown chakra. It is also thought to increase the flow of energy from the hands, so experiment with holding a labradorite palm stone before and during a Reiki session.

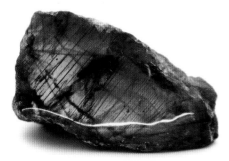

Labradorite

For Protection

Labradorite is one of the most effective stones for providing auric protection. It creates a shield of light around the energetic body, blocking negativity from entering your personal space. It is perfect for carrying or wearing if you need to spend time in toxic or emotionally draining situations. For this reason, make sure to cleanse your labradorite often.

IN A CRYSTAL GRID

Use the "Spiral" grid for this crystal (see page 122). When invoking the energy of transformation—personal, professional, spiritual—harness the power of labradorite. Use labradorite with tiger's eye for an energetic duo; their combined flash creates magic. Use a large clear quartz as the focus stone, tiger's eye as the way stones, and labradorite as the desire stones. Setting this grid signifies you're ready to light that fire, make changes, and emerge on the other side.

HEALING PROPERTIES

Mental & Emotional
For anyone who is suffering from depression, feelings of stagnancy, or a lack of passion in their life, labradorite makes for a great friend. Just as the colors of this crystal flash to life when the light strikes it perfectly, so will you find your own brilliance—let this crystal help you shine with your own wonderful light!

Spiritual
A stone of shamans and healers, it is no surprise that this crystal will help you to connect with higher spiritual realities. Labradorite enables us to see the sacred in the mundane and the amazing magic in everyday moments. Use labradorite in order to awaken your innate powers of telepathy and healing.

Physical
Labradorite is a wonderful stone to use to promote overall physical health and the balancing of systems. In particular, it can assist with neurological function, digestion, and metabolism. Labradorite can also be useful if any area of the body feels impaired or imbalanced in some way.

& As a Pairing

MOONSTONE, the feldspar cousin of labradorite, makes for a sweet and spiritually potent pairing, with each stone amplifying the energies of the other. Together they will have a powerful effect on your dreams. The flashy energy of **TIGER'S EYE** also makes a beautiful pairing—great magic can happen with these two crystals at your side.

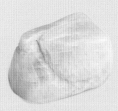

MOONSTONE

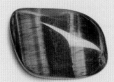

TIGER'S EYE

LARIMAR

"THE DOLPHIN STONE"

APPEARANCE
LARIMAR'S soft blue mirrors the Caribbean Sea by which it is found in only one remote area of the Dominican Republic. Swirls of light turquoise and frothy, white coloration show why it is called the "dolphin stone," although it is actually a form of blue pectolite.

MEANING
Paying homage to the sea, or *mar* in Spanish, larimar represents oceanic tranquility. In fact, it is also known as the "Atlantis stone." Strong yet gentle feminine energy heals and soothes us when we work with this natural wonder.

RARITY
Larimar is rarer by the day, as its deposits are increasingly inaccessible and scarce in the mountainous area in Barahona in the Dominican Republic where it is found.

HEALING PROPERTIES

Mental & Emotional
The ocean evokes tranquility, peacefulness, and restoration. However, that same body of water can also summon the power of a tsunami. In the same way, larimar fills us with a divine feminine energy that is both gentle and fierce. It fosters great compassion and tenderness, as well as boundaries and self-prioritization.

Spiritual
Larimar assists us in moving past difficult cycles of trauma and karmic entanglements. It allows us to remain open to receiving messages from the universe and spirit guides. Sometimes, these messages can be difficult for us to absorb and so gentle larimar can be used to soften the jagged edges.

Physical
Larimar has a cooling and soothing effect on both the emotional and the physical body. Physical conditions such as fever, inflammation, and high blood pressure can all be combated with this curative stone. Larimar can also be used to combat any issues of the neck, throat, or lymph nodes.

For Protection

Many speak of larimar's connection to the ancient, spiritually evolved civilization of Atlantis. Its discovery was prophesied by the clairvoyant Edgar Cayce, who spoke extensively from trances about this extinct civilization. It is said that by tapping into Atlantean energy, we can raise our own spiritual vibration and ward off lower, toxic frequencies.

—— In Reiki ——

Larimar is very useful on or around the neck and throat area to regulate physical or chakric imbalances. This teal-hued crystal imparts soothing energies to skin, tissues, glands, and organs, as well as to the emotional body.

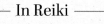

Larimar

IN A CRYSTAL GRID

Use the "Borromean Rings" grid for this crystal (see page 123). Call upon the serene vibrations of larimar to create a grid to invoke a sense of calm. Today, it's all too easy to get caught up in work stress, drama, hustle, and so on. Take a few moments and mindfully create this grid as a form of self-care. Use clear quartz as the focus stone and turquoise as the way stones—this companion crystal brings a sense of grounding. Finish the grid with larimar as the desire stones. Play soft music or chant as you create this crystal oasis of serenity.

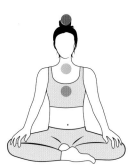

WORKING WITH THE CHAKRAS

Larimar is a preeminent throat chakra stone, enhancing areas of communication and helping us to find our inner voice. Vishuddha, the fifth chakra, which is located at the base of the throat, must be balanced and allow the free flow of energy for us to communicate our wants and needs, and also tap into our inner creativity. Larimar actually has a positive effect on all chakras from the heart up: the heart, throat, third eye, and crown chakras all respond to the soothing, spiritual energies of this oceanic gem.

IN A DAILY RITUAL

Larimar is most often found in jewelry, so daily work with it can be done with a necklace, ring, or bracelet. Having the stone right against your skin is the most effective way to absorb its healing energy. If you're working with a ring or bracelet, place them on your left, "receiving" hand and if using a necklace, try to wear it short and close to the neck.

Angels & Deities

It is speculated that larimar connects spiritually to the ancient knowledge of Atlantis.

FOR YOUR STAR SIGN

The watery sign of Pisces is a natural fit for the "dolphin stone." Pisceans will have an instant connection to larimar, as their energies are very compatible. It can help strengthen Pisceans' intuition and empathy, while enabling them to hold personal boundaries. Leo, on the other hand, connects with larimar for more healing reasons and it provides a port in the storm for this fiery sign. The calming, cooling crystal energies help combat Leo's hotheadedness.

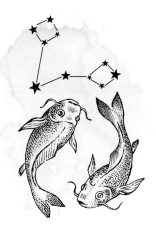

&

As a Pairing

AQUAMARINE, GRANDIDIERITE, and larimar are all beautifully compatible water stones; each complements and enhances the soothing effects of the others. Another wonderful match is **TURQUOISE,** which balances larimar's energy with an earthy and grounding vibration.

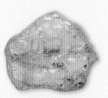

AQUAMARINE

GRANDIDIERITE

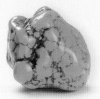

TURQUOISE

GRANDIDIERITE

"THE STONE OF THE WATER SPIRITS"

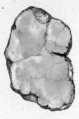

APPEARANCE

GRANDIDIERITE is a very rare, blue-green mineral, which gains its coloring from iron inclusions. It exhibits trichroism, meaning it can shift slightly between three different colors depending on which direction it is viewed. Transparent specimens are highly sought after.

MEANING

Grandidierite was discovered in 1902 in Madagascar, and named after the French explorer Alfred Grandidier. Although somewhat new to the scene, it has gained a devout following due to its potent metaphysical properties.

RARITY

Grandidierite is very rare, largely because pockets of the mineral tend to be small. For this reason, gem-quality specimens fetch incredibly high prices.

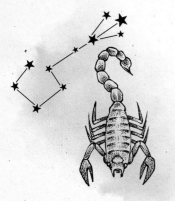

FOR YOUR STAR SIGN

Grandidierite is a water element stone, so connects with watery Pisces, Scorpio, and Cancer. Pisces will have a particularly comforting connection. Most deposits are found in Madagascar, the oldest island on the planet, so its aquatic association makes sense. The watery signs can be emotional, sensitive, and intuitive—allow grandidierite to offer guidance and protection for these qualities.

IN A DAILY RITUAL

Due to its connection to the element of water, grandidierite makes a great addition to a healing, ritual bath. This is one of the most relaxing and restorative ways to soak up some powerful crystal energy. Draw a bath and intuitively add your favorite calming elements, such as oils, herbs, or petals. Hold the grandidierite over your heart and allow its energy to wash over you.

In Reiki

Use grandidierite to stimulate the heart chakra, or any of the upper chakras. It can bring a unique, healing light to energy work sessions. If you're able to source more transparent or faceted gems, these are the most energetically potent.

Angels & Deities

There is no documented association between grandidierite and any specific deity. However, it feels strongly connected to island and water spirits.

WORKING WITH THE CHAKRAS

The avenue between the heart and throat chakras is where grandidierite comes to life. It works to balance each of these centers individually, as well as to increase the flow of energy from one to the other. The heart chakra governs issues of love and emotional well-being and the throat chakra is our center of communication—namely our ability to express ourselves and our truth. Imbalances in these areas result in relationship problems, feelings of frustration or a lack of fulfillment, depression, anxiety, reclusiveness, or loneliness. Wearing grandidierite around the neck is a great way to keep energy flowing to these areas throughout the day.

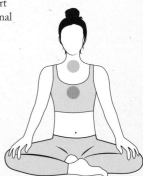

For Protection

Grandidierite creates an energetic shield of protection. It vibrates on a high frequency, keeping lower vibrational energies and intentions at bay. Raising your vibrational field will also attract energies and people on a similar level, surrounding you with light and pure, loving energy.

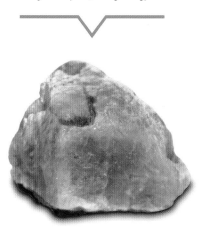

Grandidierite

IN A CRYSTAL GRID

Use the "Metatron's Cube" grid for this crystal (see page 123). Grandidierite makes an extremely powerful addition to a grid. Due to its potency and rarity, one stone will suffice, placed right at the center of the grid—your focus stone. A grid built around this gem will produce energetically intense, far-reaching results. A beautiful theme is one that sends loving energy out to all humanity; for this purpose, you'll want to use some high-vibrational stones. So, try surrounding the grandidierite with herkimer diamonds as the way stones and lemurian quartz as the desire stones.

HEALING PROPERTIES

Mental & Emotional
Grandidierite, especially in the greener tones, is a very powerful healer for the heart and our emotional well-being. It provides support to help you move through grief or heartbreak. It increases intuition, empathy, and compassion, so we are able to more effectively hold space for others, as well as ourselves.

Spiritual
Detoxifying and strengthening the aura, aligning with spirit guides, and connecting with your true purpose in life are some of the benefits of working with this mystical gem. Grandidierite removes stagnant energy from the auric field and moves us through difficult moments in life—toward the wholeness and elevation for which we're intended.

Physical
Grandidierite can be strengthening for the immune, respiratory, and nervous systems. Due to its chakric connections, it can also be used to help with heart and throat issues. Grandidierite is a good companion for anyone who is chronically unwell. As a result of this potency, even a small specimen will deliver intense healing energy.

& As a Pairing

For an incredibly powerful combination of energies, combine grandidierite with a high-vibration crystal such as **DANBURITE** or **PHENACITE**. This combination should not be used lightly, or frequently, due to its intense effects. For a softer pairing, try combining grandidierite with **LARIMAR**, a fellow water spirit stone.

DANBURITE

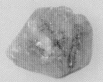

PHENACITE

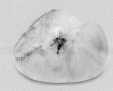

LARIMAR

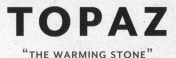

TOPAZ

"THE WARMING STONE"

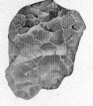

APPEARANCE

Topaz is a very hard mineral that occurs naturally in a range of colors, including blue, green, red, purple, pink, orange, and yellow, although most specimens are colorless (white topaz). Topaz is often heated or augmented to enhance the coloration.

MEANING

Topaz is one of the most ancient and legendary of all the gemstones. The name is derived from the Sanskrit word *tapas*, meaning "warmth, heat, fire"—topaz was once used to increase body heat, so helping to relieve a cold or fever.

RARITY

Imperial (or precious) topaz is the most valuable form and ranges in color from golden yellow to blush pink. Although mined globally, Brazil is one of the largest topaz producers.

IN A CRYSTAL GRID

Use the "Tripod of Life" grid for this crystal (see page 123). Small tumbled or raw pieces of topaz are relatively inexpensive. These ancient stones are incredibly versatile and work beautifully in a grid designed for increasing motivation and self-esteem. For this application we're using yellow/golden/orange topaz crystal. Place citrine in the center as the focus stone. Carnelian makes a wonderful way stone, and lastly, use topaz in the desire stone position. This combination lights up the lower chakras, creating an energy of warmth, joy, motivation, and manifestation.

FOR YOUR STAR SIGN

Topaz connects with both Sagittarius and Scorpio. Yellow topaz is a birthstone for November and blue topaz for December. For those born under the sign of Scorpio, topaz helps with emotional balance and mental clarity. It helps keep the scorpion uplifted and positive, filling their aura with its sunny, golden light. Sagittarius, the sign of the archer, responds well to stones that impart courage, tranquility, and communication, making blue topaz a perfect match.

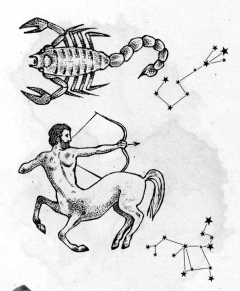

For Protection

Topaz was rumored to provide protection from magic spells, guard against enemies, and change color to indicate poisoned food. The ancient Egyptians, Hindus, Greeks, Romans, and African priests all believed topaz to have deeply protective properties.

Topaz

HEALING PROPERTIES

Mental & Emotional
Topaz imparts an energy of joyfulness, rejuvenation, compassion, and self-care. Each color yields specific benefits, yet in general it is a wonderful stone for achieving emotional clarity and inner happiness. It is no coincidence that humans have been adorning themselves with this gemstone since the dawn of civilization.

Spiritual
Topaz cleanses the aura and energy fields around the body. Metaphysically, it is a stone of purification and manifestation. It can assist with past-life recall and working through karma in this life. To achieve the deepest connection with the divine and spirit guides, choose a colorless topaz.

Physical
It has been said that topaz can be used to help improve the eyesight and also to help soothe and recharge the body in general. It was also used historically to promote calm and relaxation. Topaz can prove a helpful aid in the digestive process and also to provide relief from some eating disorders.

WORKING WITH THE CHAKRAS

Topaz's wide range of colors makes it such a versatile tool for chakric work. Clear topaz connects with the crown chakra, activating our highest spiritual selves. Blue topaz works strongly with the throat chakra, helping us to realize our inner truth and express that to those around us and the world. Pink and red topaz vibrate with the heart chakra, bringing loving energy into our daily lives. Yellow, golden, and orange topaz work with the solar plexus and sacral chakras—sparking a feeling of vitality and boosting self-confidence.

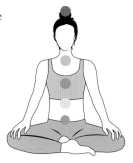

—— In Reiki ——

Topaz has a strong energy that makes it useful in energy healing. It is effective for balancing the chakras and bringing energy to stagnant or sluggish areas of the body.

Angels & Deities

Topaz is linked to both the Egyptian sun god, Ra, and Apollo, the Greek and Roman god of the sun and prophecy.

IN A DAILY RITUAL

Historically, topaz has been used to ward off darkness and negativity. In ancient times, people were instructed to wear topaz on their left arm for ultimate protection. If you find yourself under psychic or energetic attack, wear or carry some topaz on the left side of your body. Sometimes we find ourselves drained at a deep level and don't know why—try this ancient prescription!

&
As a Pairing

Combining topaz with **CITRINE** amplifies its sunny, rejuvenating energies. These two crystals were often confused with each other and, indeed, their energies are very compatible. **CARNELIAN** is similarly compatible, bringing energy down into the sacral chakra. Combining topaz with **HEMATITE** brings a grounding balance to topaz's fiery mood.

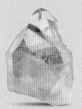

CITRINE

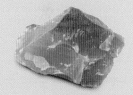

CARNELIAN

HEMATITE

K2 JASPER

"THE STONE OF ELEVATION"

APPEARANCE

K2 JASPER, also known as K2 granite, is a white granite material with orbs of blue azurite captured inside (and occasionally green touches of malachite). It is found on the K2 mountain in northern Pakistan, the second-highest peak in the world.

MEANING

Although not technically jasper, what is indisputable are the soaring spiritual vibrations of this rare stone. A geological anomaly, K2 jasper is believed to have been sent for the collective healing of humanity.

RARITY

Found in one remote region of the world, the K2 mountain, difficult mining techniques are needed to extract this stone. K2 jasper is one of the rarer pieces in a crystal toolkit.

WORKING WITH THE CHAKRAS

K2 jasper creates a very important energetic connection between the upper and the lower chakras. The granite has strong, grounding energy that speaks to muladhara, our root chakra. The azurite inclusions vibrate with the third eye and crown chakras, enhancing intuition and encouraging spiritual awakening. The result is a perfect combination of being grounded enough as an individual to truly allow a spiritual experience to occur. If either the lower or the upper chakras are blocked or imbalanced, the flow of energy will be stifled and none of the energy centers will function optimally.

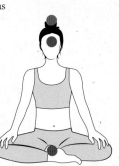

IN A DAILY RITUAL

Meditating with K2 jasper every day can produce extraordinary results in terms of mental and emotional balance, enhancing powers of intuition and furthering your spiritual journey. As K2 is both a grounding and an enlightening stone, it can be held in either hand during meditation (generally, the dominant hand is for grounding, the nondominant hand is for uplifting).

—— In Reiki ——

K2 jasper is versatile in Reiki work, as it affects different chakras and vibrational levels. It is a useful tool for the sender to attune with before an energy healing session, allowing them to ground into earthly energies and remain open to universal direction.

For Protection

Due to its molecular structure, granite embodies strength. It contains azurite's ethereal energies too, so you will feel protected by both heavenly and earthly forces when using K2 as an amulet.

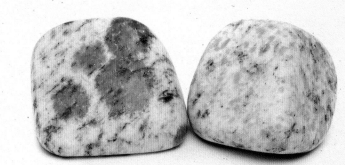

K2 jasper

IN A CRYSTAL GRID

Use the "Tripod of Life" grid for this crystal (see page 123). K2 jasper brings a unique benefit to grid work in that it has both grounding and uplifting energies. The Tripod of Life grid is ideal for anyone seeking to expand their spiritual life and practice. Use a piece of Tibetan quartz as the focus stone. This special form of quartz hails from the Himalayan mountains, neighboring K2, and imparts a similar energy. Add herkimer diamonds as the way stone and finish with K2 jasper as the desire stones—keeping the grid and your spiritual practice grounded.

Angels & Deities

Although K2 jasper is not associated with any deity, azurite, its main inclusion, is linked to Athena, the Greek goddess of wisdom and war.

HEALING PROPERTIES

Mental & Emotional

The granite component of K2 jasper provides an element of grounding, while the touches of azurite impart a higher vibration. The resulting combination is one of emotional calming, stability, and balance. Use this powerful stone to gain some insight or clarity about any situation in your life.

Spiritual

K2 jasper is a stone of spiritual enlightenment. Call upon K2 to heighten intuitive abilities, practice past-life recall, or explore the Akashic records (an unwritten compendium of all events, thoughts, words, and emotions). The grounding energy of the granite makes this a more approachable choice than other high-vibration stones.

Physical

Due to its upper chakra connection, K2 jasper can be useful in treating issues in this area, such as headaches and chronic migraines. It is generally detoxifying for the physical body and can help improve overall health. The energies of K2 promote peaceful sleep, and can also be used to help with speech problems and impediments.

FOR YOUR STAR SIGN

K2 makes a lovely match for Sagittarius—who embraces higher learning, truth seeking, and inner growth. The sign of the archer has no hesitation in shooting for the stars, and the elevating energy of this incredible stone will help that arrow find its mark. Sagittarius is never afraid to try a new venture or path in life, but that continual openness can sometimes be draining; the grounding, calming element of K2 ensures a sense of stability.

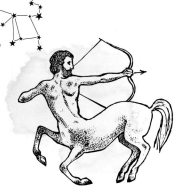

As a Pairing

K2 jasper makes an excellent companion stone for high-vibration crystals. These types of crystals can often be difficult to work with, as their energy is very intense. K2 helps to make their energy and vibration more easily assimilated. Wonderful stones for pairing are **HERKIMER DIAMOND** and **TIBETAN QUARTZ**.

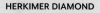

HERKIMER DIAMOND

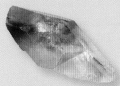

TIBETAN QUARTZ

AMETHYST

"THE STONE OF DREAMS"

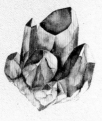

APPEARANCE
Pale lilac to dark purple in color, AMETHYST forms in prismatic crystals and attractive terminations. This semiprecious variety of quartz can be found in geodes, clusters, crystal points, cabochons, beads, and more.

MEANING
The word *amethyst* is derived from the Greek *amenthustos,* meaning "not drunken." Amethyst has a long-held association with sobriety, tranquility, peacefulness, and spiritual evolution.

RARITY
Amethyst is one of the most popular and accessible crystals. Its abundance and potency make it a wonderful stone for the beginner and crystal expert alike.

HEALING PROPERTIES

Mental & Emotional
If you find yourself weary, sad, or restless, turn to this violet gem. Amethyst is a bit of an emotional cure-all—helpful for alleviating depression, addiction issues, sleep problems, grief, and more. Amethyst is crystal balm for the tired heart and spirit.

Spiritual
Amethyst stimulates the third eye, enhancing our innate psychic ability and powers of intuition. It is also a very potent tool for meditation and dreamwork. Amethyst connects with the violet ray, a very spiritual, healing form of energy. Attuning to this crystal will help you receive guidance from higher beings.

Physical
Since the times of the ancient Greeks, it has been believed that amethyst can help prevent intoxication, and it is used today to deal with substance-abuse issues. It has a calming effect on the physical body and nervous system, and may be helpful in counteracting the effects of environmental pollution and aging.

For Protection

It is no coincidence that we often see amethyst geodes and clusters sold as decorations. The energy emitted from this beloved crystal will create a light-filled shield around the aura. Placing it around the home, or wearing it on the body, is highly recommended.

IN A DAILY RITUAL

Hold an amethyst crystal point between the eyes, over the third eye center. Then imagine an electric, violet light enveloping your whole body. Feel this protective, healing bubble of violet light all around you, then repeat the following mantra: "I am safe, I am enlightened." This particular meditation is especially helpful when you are feeling depressed or overwhelmed. It can also help if you feel that you are stagnating and in need of a lift.

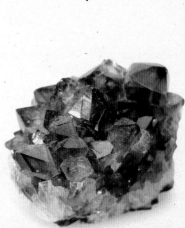

Amethyst

IN A CRYSTAL GRID

Use the "Flower of life" grid for this crystal (see page 122). Amethyst has long been associated with sobriety and letting go of harmful habits or addictions. If you feel compelled to let go of something, call on the energies of amethyst in a grid. Utilizing an array of quartz crystals will ensure an abundance of healing energy. Use a large piece of clear quartz as the focus stone, surround with citrine as the way stone for its energy of manifesting outcomes, and add amethyst as the desire stones.

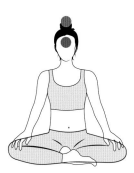

WORKING WITH THE CHAKRAS

The third eye chakra finds a great ally in amethyst crystal. *Ajna* is the Sanskrit name for this energy center, which is located just between the brows, and it translates to "beyond wisdom." It is the seat of our intuition, psychic ability, and spiritual guidance—and does, truly, exist beyond wisdom, intellect, and the thinking mind. Amethyst helps to create a connection between the third eye and crown chakras, which will really speed us along our own path of spiritual evolution.

—— In Reiki ——

Place a piece of amethyst over the third eye chakra to help you to relax into a deeper, more meditative state. This can enhance the effects of other crystals being used for healing.

Angels & Deities

As legend goes, the ancient Greek goddess Artemis saved the maiden Amethyst from Dionysus's wrath by turning her to clear crystal. His tears upon seeing her state stained her the color of wine, hence the hue.

FOR YOUR STAR SIGN

Amethyst is the official birthstone for the month of February, and it is the gemstone for the sign of Aquarius. Passionate, deep-thinking Aquarians can sometimes use a little extra stability and focus. Amethyst helps to integrate that passion and drive with a calm, grounded state of mind. These water-bearers are so busy trying to help others and change the world that they sometimes forget to sit back and take care of themselves—amethyst arrives with that gentle reminder.

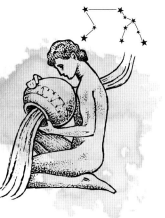

& As a Pairing

Most crystals will find a friend in amethyst. Combine with **CHRYSOPRASE** for balance; the earthiness of chrysoprase meets amethyst's ethereal energy. Most forms of quartz pair very well, but **CITRINE** in particular, being a crystal for manifestation, can help us to materialize the lofty energies and inspirations of its violet-hued cousin. Amethyst also vibrates with all varieties of quartz, specifically **OPAL** and **ROSE QUARTZ**.

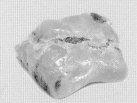

CHRYSOPRASE

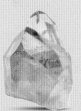

CITRINE

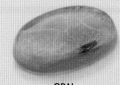

OPAL

LEPIDOLITE

"THE STONE OF TRANSITION"

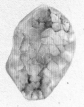

APPEARANCE

LEPIDOLITE is a lithium-bearing form of the mineral group mica and is found in shades of lavender, mauve, gray, or pink—in fact, it was originally named lilalite due to its soft coloration. The lithium can create a flaky surface appearance.

MEANING

The name *lepidolite* is derived from the Greek word *lépidos*, meaning "scale," due to its flaky texture. Also called the "grandmother stone," "peace stone," or "stone of transition" due to its nurturing, healing properties.

RARITY

Lepidolite is a relatively rare, though not unaffordable, player in the world of crystal healing. It is notably found in Brazil, Russia's Ural Mountains, and in California.

FOR YOUR STAR SIGN

The sign of Libra aligns with the soothing energies of lepidolite. Librans tend to overthink and dawdle in self-doubt; enter the calming, reassuring energy of this lavender mica. The essence of the Libran spirit is balance and harmony—and lepidolite helps those qualities to shine. Librans are naturally peaceful and sociable; their ruling planet is Venus, the signifier of love and connection. Lepidolite enhances the myriad lovely qualities of this sign of the scales, and soothes the areas that need extra attention.

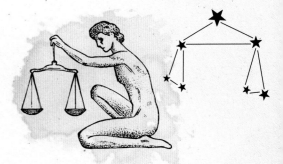

IN A CRYSTAL GRID

Use the "Spiral" grid for this crystal (see page 122). If you're drawn to dreamwork, whether this is dream recall, lucid dreaming, or just being more in tune with your subconscious, call upon the enlightening, soothing energy of lepidolite in a grid. Place a piece of amethyst in the focus stone position. Add lepidolite as the way stone and finish with charoite in the desire stone position. An extra-special touch is to add some lavender for its calming energy. Put this grid beside your bed, and keep a dream journal next to it to record any memories or insights in the morning.

Angels & Deities

Lepidolite connects with Venus, who is the Roman goddess of love.

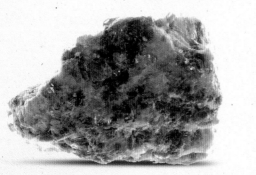

Lepidolite

For Protection

Lepidolite is known to be very effective at guarding against electromagnetic pollution. Wearing lepidolite on the body during the day will keep you safe from energetic and psychic threat. Raising your personal vibration makes you less susceptible to toxic energy.

IN A DAILY RITUAL

When meditating with lepidolite, hold the stone in your left (receiving) hand. Imagine all stress, pain, and anxiety leaving your body. Visualize violet light entering through the crown chakra at the top of your head, creating an aura of healing, protective energy all around you. As you inhale, imagine the light is entering your body. Carry this stone with you throughout the day to stay connected to that image and energy.

—— In Reiki ——

Use lepidolite anywhere on the body there is stress or tension that needs to be released. It is particularly effective for the upper chakras and in combination with other stones, depending on your specific intent.

HEALING PROPERTIES

Mental & Emotional
One of the preeminent stones for emotional healing and balance, lepidolite carries a gentle energy unlike any other. This is largely due to its high lithium content; lithium is used to make antidepressant and psychiatric medication. It is helpful for those suffering from mood swings, addiction problems, grief, or emotional instability.

Spiritual
Lepidolite is known for its powers of transformation, transition, and spiritual growth. It links strongly with the upper chakras and helps us to connect with deep, spiritual wisdom and insight. This beautiful, lilac-hued gem allows us to communicate with the higher realms and live with a heightened sense of intuition and serenity.

Physical
Lepidolite works wonders for the nervous system, easing stress and anxiety and depressive disorders. It can also be helpful for disorders of the brain due to its connection to the higher chakras. Lepidolite is known to balance hormones and for this reason is a supportive tool for women going through pregnancy or menopause.

WORKING WITH THE CHAKRAS

Lepidolite is a rare stone as it connects strongly with multiple chakras, but its preeminent association is with the crown chakra. It connects with this center of spiritual energy first, then with the third eye and heart chakras. This is in keeping with the message of lepidolite: life is all about love, and love leads to enlightenment. Use lepidolite to deepen your intuition, enhance psychic ability, and heal the heart. Empowered with lepidolite, prepare for synchronicities and signs from the universe to appear.

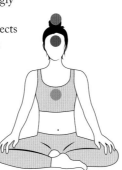

As a Pairing

CHAROITE greatly intensifies the third eye–opening energies of lepidolite when these two crystals are combined. In fact, they are often confused for one another, and this synthesis of violet energy is unparalleled for promoting psychic abilities as well as for meditation and dreamwork.

PETALITE, a high-vibration stone with a deep angelic association, creates a strong spiritual connection when it is combined with lepidolite. You can also try pairing lepidolite with **LITHIUM QUARTZ** for the ultimate uplifting and relaxing effect.

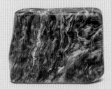

CHAROITE

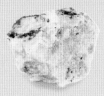

PETALITE

CHAROITE

"THE STONE OF TRANSFORMATION"

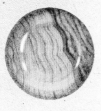

APPEARANCE

CHAROITE displays a vibrant, swirling purple coloration, with small ribbons of black and white inclusions running throughout the stone. It is also sometimes chatoyant. This rare and beautiful stone was only discovered fairly recently in the 1940s.

MEANING

Charoite is a stone of metamorphosis and transformation. The word *chary* in Russian means "magic" or "charm." This mystical stone carries an uplifting and healing vibration that supports the mind, body, and spirit.

RARITY

Charoite is a rare stone as it is only found in one location in the world—near the Chara River in eastern Siberia, after which it is named. It is still an affordable stone, however.

WORKING WITH THE CHAKRAS

Charoite, with its magical swirls of lavender, stimulates both the third eye and crown chakras. This stone can raise vibrations, connect with spirit, increase psychic ability, and access innate powers of healing. The beauty of charoite is that it allows us to access our natural gifts and abilities, so enhancing our service to those around us and humanity at large. The third eye and crown chakras, the centers of our intuition and connection to the spirit realm, receive messages that we are meant to pass on to help others, as well as ourselves.

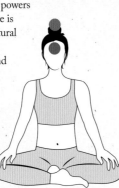

IN A DAILY RITUAL

During any time of great shifting, upheaval, or change, turn to charoite for gentle guidance and support. Rather than supplying answers or insight, the lilac-hued crystal affirms your own deep, inner knowing and provides you with the courage to trust yourself and also the stillness to find that inner voice. Meditate with charoite in your nondominant hand, or wear it on the body daily during challenging times.

—— In Reiki ——

In Reiki, charoite benefits both the sender (by enhancing intuitive abilities) and the receiver (by opening the upper chakras and protecting the aura). Place on the third eye or above the head to stimulate crown chakra opening.

For Protection

Charoite's connection to the higher spiritual realms invokes auric shielding and protection. It harnesses the guiding energy of guardian angels and spirit guides, keeping us surrounded by divine light and on our true spiritual path. It is a wonderful stone for keeping healers safe and protected from unwanted negative energy.

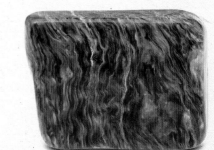

Charoite

HEALING PROPERTIES

Mental & Emotional

Charoite brings a unique clarity on many levels. It helps us to make decisions and choices from a place of love, representing the highest version of ourselves. Charoite also encourages us to trust our own instincts and innate wisdom, and to move away from fear and negativity.

Spiritual

Charoite is the perfect companion for spiritual work, as it clears the aura and enlivens the upper chakras. We all have a spiritual calling in life and charoite helps us to realize ours. It helps us to access past lives, unveil karmic lessons, and enhance energy healing work.

Physical

The peaceful energy of charoite can have a very beneficial effect on anyone struggling with ADHD, mood disorders, autism, or Asperger's syndrome. It has a detoxifying effect on the body and assists with organ function, particularly of the liver and pancreas. Charoite has also been known to regulate blood pressure.

IN A CRYSTAL GRID

Use the "Spiral" grid for this crystal (see page 122). Turn to charoite to create a beautiful grid designed to enhance and hone psychic ability. This is effective for the total beginner or someone seriously seeking to further their medium/telepathic work. Here we use only lavender-colored stones on the spiral-shaped grid template. Place an amethyst in the center of the spiral as your focus stone, to harness energy from the universe. Surround with pieces of sugilite, charoite, or any stones you feel drawn to intuitively. Place sugilite nearest the center as the way stone and use charoite as the outermost desire stones.

Angels & Deities

Connected to Sophia, the Greek goddess of spiritual wisdom, and Vac, the Hindu goddess of speech and truth.

FOR YOUR STAR SIGN

Although not a traditional birthstone or astrological assignation, charoite energy is in full effect in the darker winter months. The signs of Sagittarius and Scorpio find compatibility with the mystical charoite. It helps to calm and soothe the sign of the scorpion, letting their most beautiful qualities—passion, mental acuity, and determination—shine through. As far as the Sagittarian goes, charoite will help develop the insight they're so gifted with, as well as bring a welcome sense of balance.

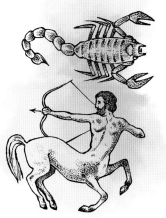

& As a Pairing

Strikingly similar in appearance, **SUGILITE** and charoite make a powerful purple duo. The transformative, spiritually potent energies of each are amplified exponentially—this is amazing for meditation or dreamwork! All that upper chakra energy can leave you feeling ungrounded, however, so try pairing charoite with jet or **BLACK TOURMALINE** to stay rooted and balanced. Pair charoite with similar-looking **LEPIDOLITE** for a synthesis of violet energy unparalleled for promoting psychic abilities.

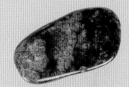

SUGILITE

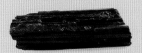

BLACK TOURMALINE

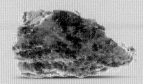

LEPIDOLITE

KUNZITE

"THE WOMAN'S STONE"

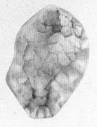

APPEARANCE
KUNZITE is the pink- or lilac-hued form of the mineral spodumene. It forms in prismatic crystals and is pleochroic, meaning its color can shift in different lighting. You may find this gem in raw form, or faceted and set in jewelry.

MEANING
Named for the famous mineralogist G. F. Kunz, kunzite represents divine love, joy, and healing energy. It is a high-vibration stone, and can bring about profound changes to your life.

RARITY
Kunzite is on the more collectible end of the spectrum, but it is possible to source rough specimens for affordable prices.

HEALING PROPERTIES

Mental & Emotional
Kunzite is a perfect choice for anyone who finds themselves embittered toward the world. It has a healing, rejuvenating effect on the heart and helps us to discover our joy in life again. Kunzite encourages playfulness and lightheartedness, and can be a useful tool for moving past old traumas.

Spiritual
Use sweet kunzite to tap into the vibration of divine love. Once we begin to accept the spiritual notion that we *are* love, and love surrounds us at all times, then we open the door to true spiritual evolution. Kunzite helps us to realize our innate ability as healers, and working with it may nudge us in that direction in our lives.

Physical
This gem is a friend to women, and can be used for relief from feminine issues and menstrual discomfort. It also assists with general heart health and can strengthen the circulatory system. If you are having physical symptoms as a result of anxiety, this is a good stone to carry or wear on the body.

For Protection

Since this crystal carries such a high vibration, it wraps the aura in protective energy. Often referred to as the "woman's stone," kunzite is a guardian stone for young girls and new mothers. Let the vibrations hold you like the hug of an old friend.

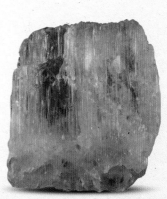

Kunzite

IN A DAILY RITUAL

Find a comfortable spot to lie down and place a piece of kunzite directly over your heart center. Close your eyes, then visualize energies of pure love swirling around you and entering through a portal where the crystal meets your body. Imagine that the kunzite crystal is a magnet for attracting love! This practice is designed to help you hold that feeling of love within your body for as long as possible.

IN A CRYSTAL GRID

Use the "Tripod of Life" grid for this crystal (see page 123). Create a grid to ensure safe travel using the spirited, protective energies of kunzite, moonstone, and smoky quartz. This can be created for yourself, your partner, your child, or anyone you hold dear, to bless them with a safe journey. Use a large smoky quartz as the central focus stone and pieces of kunzite as the way stone. Then finish with moonstone in the desire stone position. Personal touches can include a map, airplane/train ticket, or a photograph if you're sending the energy to another person. After finalizing the grid, visualize a safe departure and return.

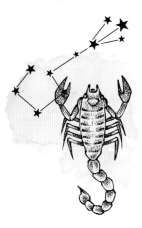

FOR YOUR STAR SIGN

Those born under the sign of the scorpion will find a friend in kunzite crystal. Scorpio's intensity can be both a blessing and a curse, and this soothing stone will help cool the waters. Scorpios are loyal companions and take their relationships very seriously; if they are scorned or heartbroken, learning to trust again can be a challenge. Kunzite helps to reopen and reenergize a weary heart, making love and trust possible again.

Angels & Deities

Kunzite is associated with Venus, the ancient Roman goddess of love, sex, beauty, and fertility.

——— In Reiki ———

Use kunzite on any parts of the body that appear to be holding stress. It emits a powerful, calming energy that is beneficial for any hands-on energy work.

WORKING WITH THE CHAKRAS

Kunzite makes an important link between the heart chakra and the crown chakra, aligning our emotional center and higher mind. We are more inclined to receive deep, spiritual insights when our heart center feels stable and emotionally secure. The energy also flows both ways, as our experience with divine love through the crown chakra opening will bring strength and balance to the heart. These two chakras working in tandem will open us up empathically and increase altruistic desires. The spiritual lesson that kunzite imparts is that love begets more love!

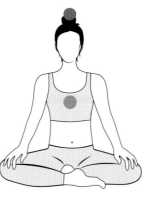

As a Pairing

HIDDENITE is the yellow-green variety of spodumene, and makes a powerful pairing with its lilac-hued cousin, kunzite. Their two energies compound each other, amplifying the effects of each. **MOONSTONE** also makes a wonderful crystal companion, which increases the protective energies of kunzite, especially during times of travel.

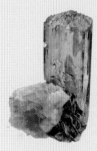

HIDDENITE

MOONSTONE

ROSE QUARTZ

"THE STONE OF UNCONDITIONAL LOVE"

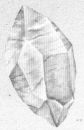

APPEARANCE

ROSE QUARTZ ranges from very pale pink to a deep, reddish hue. It can be opaque or translucent, and is generally found in tumbled, rough, or carved from. Occasionally, strands of rutile will be present, producing the appearance of a glowing "star" within the crystal.

MEANING

In ancient myths, rose quartz was said to have been formed when the goddess Aphrodite brushed against thorns while running to save her lover, Adonis. It has always symbolized the power of love, renewal, and vitality.

RARITY

An abundant and affordable variety of quartz crystal. Crystallized rose quartz, with individual terminations, is the rarest and most precious form of this beloved stone.

HEALING PROPERTIES

Mental & Emotional

The ultimate stone for all matters of the heart is undeniably rose quartz. Emanating a gentle, love-filled energy, it soothes our emotions like no other. This crystal helps us move past old trauma, particularly from childhood.

Spiritual

Rose quartz embodies love above all else. It carries divine feminine energy, and can connect us with our soul's true purpose in life. When worn on the body or used in meditation, it works to cleanse the aura of any toxic, negative energy or attachments.

Physical

Unsurprisingly, rose quartz is very healing for the physical heart, as well as the circulatory system. It has also been used since ancient Egyptian times in beauty treatments to create a youthful, more refreshed appearance.

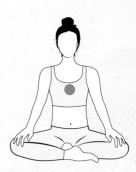

WORKING WITH THE CHAKRAS

Some people claim rose quartz is the single most important crystal for working with anahata, the heart chakra. It can be beneficial on some level for all the chakras, but the heart center is definitely the most affected by rose quartz energy. *Anahata*, in Sanskrit, roughly translates as "unhurt, unstruck, unbeaten." Imagine living life with a fully open heart, one that is not jaded from heartbreak of the past. That is what the power of rose quartz can release: a freedom from fear and bitterness…a belief in the divine possibility of each new day, knowing you are surrounded by an unending, universal love.

IN A DAILY RITUAL

Rose quartz face masks have been found buried in ancient Egyptian tombs, so this crystal's association with beauty and self-care is nothing new. One fun and rejuvenating activity is to make rose quartz water. Simply fill a jar with some filtered or spring water and a few rose quartz stones of your choice, then leave this outside in sunlight or moonlight for twelve hours. Drink the water as a special tonic or use it in facial mists, alone or with a combination of your favorite oils.

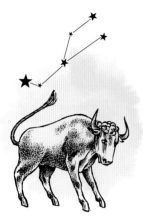

FOR YOUR STAR SIGN

Although not a traditional birthstone, rose quartz is beneficial for those born under the sign of Taurus. Taurus is ruled by the planet Venus, the celestial body associated with love and beauty. Individuals born under this sign often need a reminder to love themselves first, which is a particular energetic benefit of rose quartz. Stubborn, often hot-headed Taureans are soothed by this gem.

IN A CRYSTAL GRID

Use the "Flower of Life" grid for this crystal (see page 122). Rose quartz makes a potent addition to any crystal grid and is quite versatile within the grid itself. It is recommended for any grid built around the themes of love, forgiveness, or healing. You can create a grid to empower the heart chakra, using the Flower of Life template. Choose a large piece of rose quartz to act as the focus stone. Flesh out the grid with pieces of rhodochrosite, raw emerald, morganite, or green calcite. Select the way and desire stones intuitively; these crystals are interchangeable. I like to add some rose petals to heart-based grids for the extra sweet energy that they bring.

Angels & Deities

Rose quartz strongly resonates with goddess energy—the Greek Aphrodite and Egyptian goddess Isis are two ancient connections.

——— In Reiki ———

In Reiki healing, rose quartz is a universally potent tool. In addition to body placement, one beautiful method of utilizing this rosy gem is to surround the receiver with it. Encircle the body with pieces of rose quartz to create a deeply peaceful, love-filled space for healing to take place.

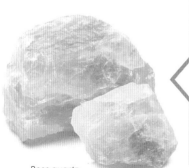

Rose quartz

For Protection

Rose quartz has always been a source of protection for women, especially pregnant women and mothers. The vibration is soft enough that it can be used with babies and very young children. Carrying a strong goddess energy, this stone also helps us to create boundaries—but from a place of gentle strength.

& As a Pairing

You can combine rose quartz with almost any crystal to create a softer, gentler energy. It is compatible with all varieties of quartz crystal, including **CLEAR QUARTZ**. Favorite companions to amplify the heart-healing effects are **EMERALD** and **RHODOCHROSITE**. Rose quartz can also be combined with **OPAL**, **MORGANITE**, and **MOLDAVITE** for powerful results. The effects of moldavite can often be too intense to process fully, but rose quartz can help to soften that experience, allowing us to receive and assimilate its full, transformative benefits.

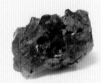

EMERALD

RHODOCHROSITE

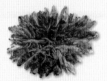

MOLDAVITE

RHODOCHROSITE

"THE STONE OF THE COMPASSIONATE HEART"

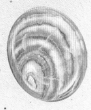

APPEARANCE

RHODOCHROSITE is most commonly light pink to raspberry red in color, and marked by bands of color throughout. It is usually found alongside natural deposits of silver. Being a softer gemstone, it is sometimes difficult to set in jewelry, but is an excellent choice for meditation or energy work.

MEANING

The word *rhodochrosite* is derived from the Greek for "rose color." The Incas, upon discovering deposits of this rose-hued crystal, believed it to be the blood of deceased royalty.

RARITY

Generally speaking, specimens of rhodochrosite are easily obtained and range from quite affordable to those that sell for "collector" prices. However, well-formed crystals are rather rare and can fetch higher prices.

IN A DAILY RITUAL

The beauty of rhodochrosite lies in its ability to help us see, love, and accept ourselves, often through inner-child healing work. A deeply effective practice involves meditating with a photograph of yourself as a child—just use your intuition to choose one that evokes an emotional response. Hold the photo in your right hand and a piece of rhodochrosite in your left. Look at the child in the photo and summon all the protective, loving, tender emotion you would have if he or she were standing before you. Keep the crystal in your pocket over the next few days, and call upon those feelings of love when self-doubt, criticism, or inadequacy emerge.

FOR YOUR STAR SIGN

Those born under the sign of Scorpio will find a friend in rhodochrosite. Scorpios can be brilliant, quick-tempered, and forceful. The sign of the scorpion is well balanced by the rosy rhodochrosite crystal. The calming vibrations can bring ease and peacefulness to Scorpios, allowing their many inherent gifts to shine properly. Scorpios can achieve nearly anything they set their mind to, and rhodochrosite helps to make the path to that end goal more pleasant and palatable for them and those around them.

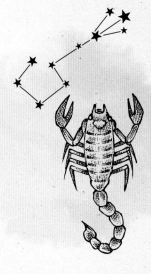

WORKING WITH THE CHAKRAS

Unsurprisingly, this rosy crystal has a strong connection with the heart chakra, but it works just as effectively with the solar plexus chakra. Rhodochrosite bolsters our self-confidence and self-love, opening our hearts to fully receive love from others. If you are seeking to overcome past trauma or destructive habits or mindsets, focus the stone on your solar plexus. Once progress has been made and you feel ready to move on, visualize drawing the energy from that area up to the heart center. Use your crystal as a tool to help draw the energy upward!

—— In Reiki ——

Placing rhodochrosite over the heart chakra is the most common use for it in energy healing practices. To encourage self-esteem, place rhodochrosite over the solar plexus. To activate creativity, you may center it on the sacral chakra. Practice making energetic connections between all three chakras to feel the ultimate benefit.

For Protection

Rhodochrosite encourages us to become our own fiercest protectors by reminding us that we are deserving of love, support, and unconditional kindness. Why would we accept any less for ourselves than we would want for our dearest friend? This pink friend bolsters our self-confidence and self-love, ensuring we accept no less than we deserve.

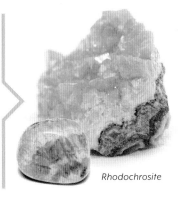

Rhodochrosite

Angels & Deities

The Chinese goddess Guanyin, mother of compassion and mercy, claims a strong connection to the sweet rhodochrosite.

IN A CRYSTAL GRID

Use the "Spiral" grid for this crystal (see page 122). We often find ourselves stuck or suffering as adults because we need to heal our inner child. If you feel compelled to do this, creating a grid with rhodochrosite can be a helpful step toward healing. Put a rose quartz in the focus stone position. Inner-child trauma is usually held in the sacral chakra, so put pieces of carnelian in the way stone position. Finish your grid with rhodochrosite as the desire stones. Feel free to add a photograph of yourself as a child.

HEALING PROPERTIES

Mental & Emotional
Are you looking to connect with your inner child? Look no further, as rhodochrosite is the perfect tool for realizing your innate innocence and unbridled joy. Use this heart-centered stone to connect with ultimate love and compassion for yourself, which will allow you to direct that loving-kindness toward the outside world as a whole.

Spiritual
The energy of rhodochrosite is more of a gentle kiss than a strong blow. Its energetic softness can make deep, spiritual lessons more palatable. This gem allows us to reform any long-held negative feelings about ourselves, which may hinder present-day relationships and our ability to connect deeply with others.

Physical
Rhodochrosite is healing for both the nervous and the circulatory systems. The manganese present in this mineral may be helpful with tissue repair, bone growth, and issues with the skin.

& As a Pairing

Rhodochrosite pairs well with its sister stone, **ROSE QUARTZ**. At times, the work we are doing with rhodochrosite—particularly inner-child healing work—can be difficult, and the addition of rose quartz helps soften our journey. Additionally, **CARNELIAN** makes a beautiful pairing with rhodochrosite. Often, we find our hearts blocked or not fully open, and carnelian helps us to discover our true "self," which must feel secure and precious before we can offer our hearts to anyone else.

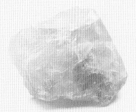

ROSE QUARTZ

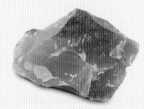

CARNELIAN

MORGANITE

"THE GENTLE HEART STONE"

APPEARANCE

MORGANITE is part of the beryl family—a mineral group that includes aquamarine and emerald. It is typically pink to pinkish-orange in color due to the presence of manganese. Morganite's color appears to change when it is viewed from different angles.

MEANING

Morganite is associated with divine love and the energy of the heart. It helps us to heal old wounds and move past trauma, while at the same time wrapping us in the loving energy of the universe.

RARITY

In terms of geological abundance, morganite is rarer than diamond. High-quality, faceted specimens fetch high prices, but rough forms are more accessible.

FOR YOUR STAR SIGN

Although not considered a traditional birthstone, the cooling energy of morganite is particularly beneficial for those born under the sign of Taurus. Taurus is ruled by Venus, the goddess of love, which makes this gentle heart stone a calming companion for the passionate children of Taurus. Those born under the sign of Cancer may also benefit from the tranquil energy of morganite.

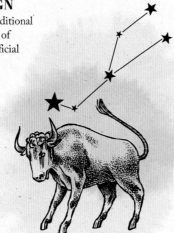

—— In Reiki ——

Place morganite directly over the heart for a deeply healing experience. Focus on the warm embrace of love that surrounds you and allow it to free you from any trauma or pain you have been experiencing.

Angels & Deities

Morganite is a wonderful stone for angelic connection and is closely associated with the guardian angels Hariel, Hahahel, Ariel, and Mihael. It is also connected to Astarte, the ancient warrior goddess of love and fertility.

For Protection

When used as a talisman, morganite can guide us away from old habits or negative behavioral patterns and give us the strength to trust our inner compass. It directs the heart to its true spiritual path, allowing us to interact with the world from a place of compassion, joy, and openness.

Morganite

IN A CRYSTAL GRID

Use the "Flower of Life" grid for this crystal (see page 122) to signify the heart blossoming. Morganite is a powerful stone in a grid, ideal for heart healing, opening, and honoring. When the heart is broken, resentful, or afraid to open fully, we suffer in nearly every area of our life. Use rose quartz as the focus stone to imbue the grid with sweet energy. Use lithium quartz points as the way stone and morganite as the desire stones. Then light a candle to honor the brave work you are doing so well.

IN A DAILY RITUAL

Hold the morganite in your left hand, or place over the heart, and visualize the flow of unconditional love entering your body from all around you. Visualize it filling your chest and gradually your entire body with a soft, humming light. Know that in this light you are safe, and held. In moments of tension or fear, remember this vision of light, and know that it is always within you.

HEALING PROPERTIES

Mental & Emotional

Morganite heals and energizes the heart, creating a sense of calm by encouraging a connection with the divine energy of the universe. It lets us release attachments to ideas, relationships, and thoughts that no longer serve us. Wearing or working with this stone fills us with the knowledge that we are loved—and capable of love in turn.

Spiritual

This stone opens and balances energy through the heart chakra, infusing our aura with lightness of spirit. This gentle gem is a token for manifestation, encouraging us to create the fulfilling life we deserve. When our hearts are open and our spirits connected to divine love, we may contribute toward the greater universal good.

Physical

Morganite strengthens the heart and is also a wonderful crystal medicine for the nervous system, thyroid, and libido. It has a detoxifying effect on our physical bodies and is a particular friend to women and girls.

WORKING WITH THE CHAKRAS

Anahata, the heart chakra, is where morganite truly shines. The Sanskrit word *anahata* roughly translates as "unhurt, unstruck, unbeaten," and the greatest gift of morganite is that it allows us to love and live as if we have never been brokenhearted. Its gentle, soothing presence can help us overcome trauma and grief, emerging on the other side ready to give and receive unconditional love. When our heart chakra is balanced, it allows the free flow of energy. This in turn empowers us to interact with the world in a loving and authentic way.

As a Pairing

If you are working with the heart chakra, trauma, or emotional healing, pair morganite with **ROSE QUARTZ** or **LITHIUM QUARTZ**. To enhance heart-based energies, the combination of morganite with **MALACHITE** is unmatched. Morganite always enjoys the company of other beryl minerals such as **AQUAMARINE** and **EMERALD**, as their energies vibrate at very compatible frequencies.

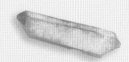

LITHIUM QUARTZ

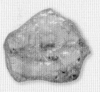

AQUAMARINE

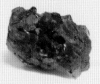

EMERALD

LITHIUM QUARTZ

"THE STONE OF CALMING ENERGY"

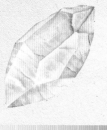

APPEARANCE

LITHIUM QUARTZ is a variety of quartz crystal with inclusions of the mineral lithium, ranging from pale pink to lavender to dark mauve. Often seen in prismatic crystal points, crystal clusters, or in tumbled form.

MEANING

Much like the antidepressant drug of the same name, this stone is synonymous with uplifting, healing, calming energy. It may assist with depression, anxiety, and mood swings.

RARITY

As a variety of quartz—the second most abundant mineral in the earth's crust after feldspar—a lithium crystal should be moderately available and affordable.

IN A CRYSTAL GRID

Use the "Flower of Life" grid for this crystal (see page 122). Call upon the soothing, uplifting energies of lithium quartz in a crystal grid if you're suffering from depression, grief, or anxiety. All forms of quartz make wonderful focus stones, and this variety is no exception. Place a large point or cluster of lithium quartz in the center of the grid. Use lepidolite as the way stone and finish with amethyst in the desire stone position. Meditate over this grid, taking deep, healing breaths, and allow its calming energies to wash over you.

FOR YOUR STAR SIGN

Lithium quartz is beneficial for every sign of the zodiac, but those born under Aquarius will find they have a particular connection with this calming crystal. Aquarians are so busy trying to fix the world and solve everyone's problems, they often forget to fill their own cup. Lithium quartz crystal reminds the water-bearer to take care of their own needs first. It's also exhausting trying to do it all—this crystal helps you to pause, relax, recharge, and practice some self-care.

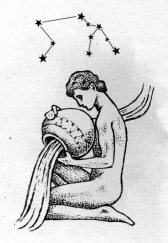

For Protection

Lithium quartz is a very effective stone to carry, either in your pocket or, even better, in jewelry form. It raises the vibration of the wearer, so destructive, toxic energies cannot attach to the aura. The longer you work with this lilac-hued beauty, the more you will attract brighter, more positive energy into your life.

Lithium quartz

HEALING PROPERTIES

Mental & Emotional
Lithium quartz has a profoundly calming, restorative effect on our emotional state. It can help us to work through repressed grief or trauma, offering gentleness and grace as we traverse these painful paths. Anyone who suffers from depression, anxiety, addiction, or mental health issues will find a friend in lithium quartz.

Spiritual
Lithium quartz carries an uplifting vibration that promotes the flow of positive energy throughout the body and auric field. On a spiritual level, it is a great teacher as it seeks to show us that we are separate from what ails us. We are pure, divine love, simply having a human experience.

Physical
This stone has a calming effect on the whole physical body and specifically the nervous system. If you are prone to stress, carry a piece in your pocket or on the body.

WORKING WITH THE CHAKRAS

Lithium quartz is effective when working with all chakras. Its soothing, balancing energy is a supreme tool in energy healing work. However, it has a particular affinity with the heart and third eye chakras. Use lithium quartz over anahata, the heart, when muscles feel weary or stressed. Focusing it over ajna, the third eye, may enhance powers of telepathy, intuition, or shamanic work.

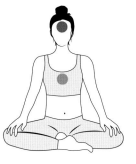

—— In Reiki ——

Use lithium quartz wherever there is tension in the physical or energetic body. Tumbled stones or palm stones are wonderful tools for bodywork, imparting a general sense of healing and relaxation.

Angels & Deities

Lithium quartz brings you into alignment with your own personal guardian angels.

IN A DAILY RITUAL

A ritual bath is the perfect setting to soak up all the soothing energies of lithium crystals. Draw a bath, add some lavender oil, and whatever relaxes your spirit—maybe rose or calendula petals. Select every element mindfully, as if you're preparing a special gift (you are!). Place lithium quartz tumbled stones, point(s), or a crystal cluster in the bathwater or on the edge of the tub.

As a Pairing

Pair lithium quartz with **LEPIDOLITE**, a lithium-based mineral, for the ultimate uplifting and relaxing effect. Often, when we are working with lithium quartz, difficult emotions and old wounds can be brought to the surface—use **MORGANITE** to help ease this process.

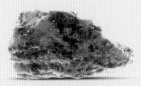

LEPIDOLITE

MORGANITE

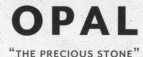

OPAL

"THE PRECIOUS STONE"

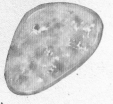

APPEARANCE

Technically not a crystal, OPAL falls into the mineraloid category. Opal is composed of silicon dioxide and water, making it amorphous. It has been revered for millennia due to its flashy, mesmerizing plays of color.

MEANING

The word "opal" is originally derived from the Sanskrit *upala*, meaning "precious stone." Although there are many different forms of opal, here we will be looking in detail at precious opal.

RARITY

Opal is at the more costly end of the spectrum and mostly features in fine jewelry. Black opal is very rare and valuable.

WORKING WITH THE CHAKRAS

Opal claims a connection to the higher chakras, specifically the crown and third eye. However, it can be used on any chakra if necessary due to its multicolored light. It has been revered as a stone of prophecy since ancient times, lifting the veil between the physical and psychic realms. Hold your opal over the third eye during meditation to increase psychic awareness, or over the top of the head to invite divine light and wisdom down into the crown chakra. The higher chakras are the gateway between our thinking minds and a deeper, spiritual realm of existence—use opal as your door between the two.

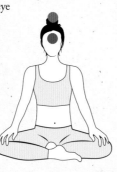

IN A DAILY RITUAL

One of the most common places you'll find opal is in jewelry, so feel free to use a piece of jewelry or a loose specimen for the following meditation. Allow the opal to be your point of focus and gaze into its flashing iridescence for a few moments. Repeat to yourself: "I am open to the magic of the universe." What it took for the universe to form this glistening opal was nothing short of magic; the same goes for you.

—— In Reiki ——

Use opal wherever there is a blockage in the body, physical or energetic. Due to its water content and uplifting vibration, it has the ability to break up and lend fluidity to any areas of stagnation.

For Protection

Opal may provide emotional protection since it can distract energies, in much the same way that it "distracts" beams of light to create its signature rainbow flash. It repairs and strengthens the auric field, amplifying our connection to the divine and warding off negative energies.

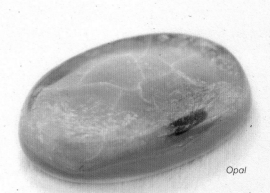

Opal

IN A CRYSTAL GRID

Use the "Spiral" grid for this crystal (see page 122). It is nearly impossible to gaze upon an opal without feeling at least a hint of magic, wonder, and joy. Harness this incredible quality by creating a grid to enhance those feelings: joyfulness, childlike wonder, humbling awe…things that we too often forget to make time for in our busy adult lives. Choose a beautiful piece of clear quartz for the focus stone. Place opal in the way stone position and alternate rose quartz and amethyst in a repeating pattern to make up the desire stones. You'll never want to take this thing of beauty apart!

Angels & Deities

Opal is said to have formed when the tears of Zeus hit the ground. It is also associated with the Roman goddess Ops, the wife of Saturn.

HEALING PROPERTIES

Mental & Emotional
The way the light dances off an opal makes it no surprise that this gem encourages spontaneity, creativity, and optimism. It brings a sense of magic and wonder into the everyday. Often referred to as a stone of amplification, opal has the ability to enhance whatever we are directing our energy toward, whether negative or positive.

Spiritual
Opal fills the aura with a divine light! It raises the frequency of the user/wearer, allowing us to communicate more clearly with our guardian angels and spirit guides. Opal is a karmic stone, representing the idea that whatever we put out into the universe, we receive back in turn, several times over.

Physical
Due to the high water content of opal, it can be helpful if you struggle with water retention issues. Additionally, it has a long-held association with the eyes, so can be beneficial for vision problems.

FOR YOUR STAR SIGN

Opal is regarded as the birthstone for the month of October, along with black tourmaline. Thus, lucky Libra can claim a special connection to this magical gem. Librans tend to be peace-loving, to the extent of forfeiting their own needs so as not to cause any disharmony. Opal fills the wearer with a sense of confidence and decisiveness, bringing this star sign into alignment with their true wants and needs in life. Librans have an innate attraction to things of rare beauty and opulence, making this fiery gemstone a true match.

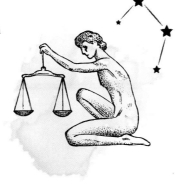

As a Pairing

Try pairing opal with **BLACK OBSIDIAN** to bring out the best in this flashy gem. The obsidian, also a mineraloid, helps create a shield around the aura while you dance in the ethereal heights of opal's energy. Combining with **PEARL** opens up dazzling crown chakra energy. Opal also vibrates with all varieties of quartz, specifically **AMETHYST** and **ROSE QUARTZ.**

BLACK OBSIDIAN

PEARL

AMETHYST

ROSE QUARTZ

FLUORITE

"THE GENIUS STONE"

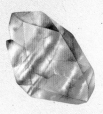

APPEARANCE

FLUORITE is in the halide family, and is one of the most colorful minerals in the world. It forms in cubes and octahedrons, and can be found in the colors blue, purple, pink, green, yellow, clear, black, or a combination thereof.

MEANING

Fluorite was the first mineral to be categorized as fluorescent. The word "fluorite" is derived from the Latin *fluere*, which means "to flow," as it was often used as flux. It is known as the "genius stone" due to its ability to enhance mental abilities.

RARITY

You'll likely find fluorite anywhere crystals are sold, with only rarer colors and formations fetching higher prices.

WORKING WITH THE CHAKRAS

Each color of fluorite carries its own specific chakric association, but all fluorite is universally balancing for the chakra system as a whole. Purple and clear fluorite both work with the crown chakra and our highest spiritual journeying; purple also opens the third eye and psychic ability. Blue crystals speak to the throat chakra, while green fluorite is a treat for the heart chakra. Yellow crystals speak to the solar plexus chakra and our self-will, while rainbow fluorite works to synergize all of the chakras together.

IN A DAILY RITUAL

Fluorite is the perfect stone for the practice of meditation, which can often be the gateway to a true spiritual awakening. The energy of fluorite assists with the very thing that so many of us often struggle with when we sit down to meditate: quieting the overactive mind. Try sitting with fluorite once a day, just for a few minutes at a time to start with—practicing that one simple, and yet oh-so-difficult, act.

—— In Reiki ——

Use fluorite for overall purification of energy, for the receiver and the sender at the same time. Use in body layouts, or just place a large specimen in the room during healing sessions to keep the energy clear.

For Protection

Raising our vibrational frequency makes us less susceptible to psychic attack. Fluorite creates a shield around the aura, surrounding us with divine light, but it also raises our powers of intuition so we are less prone to entertain potentially harmful people or situations.

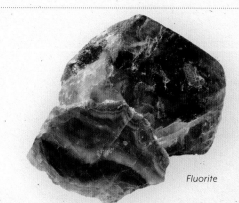

Fluorite

FOR YOUR STAR SIGN

Those born under the sign of Capricorn will find that they have a true ally in fluorite—orderliness, balance, and organization unite the energies of Capricorn and fluorite. Pisceans will also find that they benefit greatly from working with this spirited gem. Pisces is a very intuitive, spiritual astrological sign. But Pisceans can sometimes be carried away and swept along by emotionality. Fluorite can be used by Pisceans to help them keep their minds focused and ensure their emotions are kept in proportion.

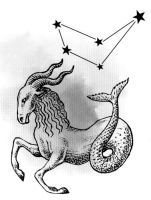

HEALING PROPERTIES

Mental & Emotional

Fluorite is associated with the mind, as it balances and coordinates both hemispheres of the brain, so they work optimally—on their own and in conjunction. It can help with brain fog, indecisiveness, and indifference. Bringing emotional clarity and balance, it allows us to identify our feelings and address our needs accordingly.

Spiritual

All colors of fluorite are very psychically cleansing, ridding the aura of stagnant, toxic energies. It raises the vibration of the individual, opening us to deeper spiritual insights. Fluorite not only helps us uncover these spiritual truths, it then assists us in mentally assimilating the information and carrying it in everyday life.

Physical

Unsurprisingly, fluorite is very supportive of brain function and health. It can assist those who are prone to headaches or memory loss. Fluorite is strengthening for the nervous and immune systems, bettering our overall physical health.

IN A CRYSTAL GRID

Use the "Tripod of Life" grid for this crystal (see page 123). Use fluorite in a grid designed to detoxify your energetic body. Occasionally we may find ourselves feeling "cluttered" with other people's energy—unavoidable in the workplace or family situations—and compelled to do an energetic cleanse! Use a large piece of clear quartz as the focus stone, fluorite (any color or shape) as the way stone, and black obsidian as the desire stones. The obsidian keeps us energetically protected as we purge any negativity.

Angels & Deities

Fluorite is associated with the Hindu goddess Vac, who ruled over the spoken word.

& As a Pairing

Fluorite and **BLACK OBSIDIAN** make a supreme duo for energetic protection. If you find yourself under psychic attack, carry these stones in your pocket or wear them on the body at all times. Combine fluorite with **LAPIS LAZULI** to enhance its powers of mental clarity and intellectual elevation.

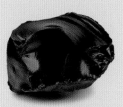

BLACK OBSIDIAN

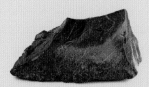

LAPIS LAZULI

BLACK TOURMALINE

"THE SHIELDING STONE"

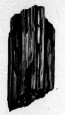

APPEARANCE
BLACK TOURMALINE is pitch-black in color and has visible striations running through it. An incredibly hard mineral, some form of inclusion is usually present. It is also slightly pleochroistic, meaning the color will change slightly when the crystal is turned in the light.

MEANING
Also known as schorl, black tourmaline is one of the preeminent stones for energetic shielding and protection. It is both pyroelectric and piezoelectric, meaning it can produce and hold an electrical charge.

RARITY
Black tourmaline, the most abundant form of tourmaline, is relatively affordable and not difficult to find, making it an easy addition to your crystal toolkit.

HEALING PROPERTIES

Mental & Emotional
Black tourmaline offers profound assistance when you are trying to combat anxiety, stress, and depression. It constantly works to cleanse the emotional body of negativity and any toxic attachments. In addition, its ability to ground you into the balancing energy of the earth cannot be overstated.

Spiritual
Black tourmaline is highly effective at deflecting and removing negative energies from the aura. It creates a strong energetic connection to the earth, keeping us grounded for any spiritual work. Think of it as the warrior who keeps us guarded, freeing us to deepen our connection with the divine and our innermost selves.

Physical
On every level, including the physical plane, you can benefit greatly from wearing or working with black tourmaline on a daily basis. It can increase energy levels and physical vitality. It has a detoxifying effect on the whole body. It is particularly useful for the lungs, helping to calm the effects of pneumonia and bronchitis.

IN A DAILY RITUAL
Using black tourmaline in your living space is a great way to utilize its protective and transformative powers on a daily basis. After cleansing your stones (in water or on top of selenite are both great methods), place a piece in the four corners of your room or house. This creates a passive way to purify the energy that you're coming into contact with throughout the day. These crystals are doing some heavy work, so be sure to cleanse and charge them frequently!

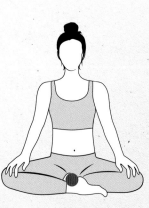

WORKING WITH THE CHAKRAS
Black tourmaline is a *must-have* crystal tool for any lower chakra work, particularly the root chakra. The Sanskrit word for this first chakra is *muladhara*, which translates as the words for "root" and "support." Muladhara is the energy center that grounds us into the earth, and must be in balance for any other higher chakra to function properly. The root chakra governs our sense of emotional and physical safety, and black tourmaline rises to the challenge of providing a stabilizing effect in those areas.

IN A CRYSTAL GRID

Use the "Vesica Piscis" grid for this crystal (see page 122). There is something alluring about combining crystals with opposite energies. So, create a yin-and-yang grid to bring grounding to a spiritual practice. Use clear quartz as the focus stone, black tourmaline as the way stone, and selenite as the desire stones. Crown chakra–opening clear quartz and selenite make the perfect match with black tourmaline's root chakra–based energy.

FOR YOUR STAR SIGN

Those born under the sign of Libra are lucky to claim black tourmaline as their astrological match. Librans, with their inner sense of balance and stability, gravitate toward those same qualities in this powerful stone. Additionally, they find great comfort in the stress-relieving qualities of black tourmaline, as the intensity of their nature can, at times, feel overwhelming. Capricorns also have an energetic compatibility with this stone. Capricorns, with their fierce determination and seriousness, may find themselves feeling calmer, as well as more able to focus and receive criticism with this crystal heavy-hitter in their corner (or pocket).

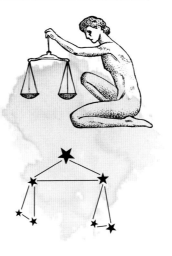

For Protection

The name black tourmaline is almost synonymous with "protection." Due to its incredible physical and metaphysical benefits, it creates a shield of protection like no other. Black tourmaline can even help to block electromagnetic frequency and radiation, a very helpful quality in our present-day world.

Angels & Deities

Black tourmaline has a connection to the Arabic goddess Manat, who was associated with death, destiny, and faith.

—— In Reiki ——

Black tourmaline is ideal to use wherever there is an imbalance or pain in the body, as it works beautifully to restore harmony in the physical body and remove toxicity.

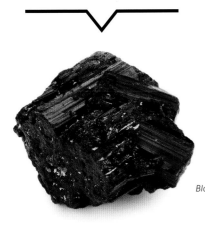

Black tourmaline

& As a Pairing

Pair tourmaline with **SELENITE** or **PHENACITE** for an unbeatable combination: both grounding and uplifting (as a bonus, the selenite keeps the tourmaline cleansed and ready to work). Tourmaline works well with other grounding stones like **HEMATITE** and **DRAVITE** to amplify energy. Combined with **MALACHITE**, tourmaline helps maintain a safe heart-space and boundaries and creates a matchless protective energy with **SMOKY QUARTZ**. Use black tourmaline with **CHAROITE** to stay rooted and balanced during upper chakra energy work.

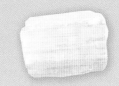

SELENITE

MALACHITE

SMOKY QUARTZ

SHUNGITE

"THE MIRACLE STONE"

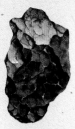

APPEARANCE

SHUNGITE is a black, carbon-based mineral with a metallic appearance. Its origins are a bit of a mystery, but we know it is over two billion years old and contains molecules called fullerenes. These are said to be highly protective and purifying, as well as antioxidant and even antibacterial.

MEANING

In crystal energy, shungite—which contains nearly all the elements of the periodic table—is synonymous with protection. The name shungite is derived from the Russian village of Shunga, where it is largely found.

RARITY

Found in just a few places outside of northeastern Russia, this miraculous mineral is somewhat rare, but is nonetheless available at a range of prices.

WORKING WITH THE CHAKRAS

Shungite connects to the lower chakras and specifically to the root chakra. It imparts a deep sense of grounding, connecting us to steady, healing earth energy. It is essential to keep muladhara, the root chakra, balanced and free-flowing, or all of the other chakras may suffer. This chakra governs our survival instinct and sense of security in the world; it must be working effectively before any kind of spiritual work can be attempted. Wearing shungite on the body or carrying a stone in the pocket can help to bring grounding energy to our first chakra throughout the day.

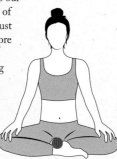

IN A DAILY RITUAL

Making shungite water has been practiced in Russia for many centuries. The water was used to treat warriors coming out of battle and there is a lake near the natural shungite deposit from which people can drink directly without needing to treat the water first. Placing shungite stones at the bottom of a water pitcher for twenty-four hours will remove many of its impurities.

IN A CRYSTAL GRID

Use the "Square" grid for this crystal (see page 123). Shungite serves many purposes in a grid. Its primary effects are protection and purification, but due to its conductivity, it can also amplify those of any surrounding stones. To make the most use of its qualities, create a square-shaped grid for strength and protection. Choose smoky quartz as the focus stone. Place shungite in the way stone position and surround with black obsidian. This is an unbeatable combination to keep you safe, grounded, and secure. Feel free to augment with any other crystals that feel suitable for your situation.

For Protection

Use shungite to block you from the pervasive presence of electromagnetic frequencies, as well as different levels of negative energy. Its molecular makeup places this mineral among the most protective and shielding stones that you can use.

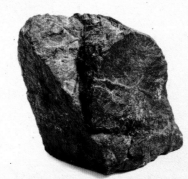

Shungite

In Reiki

Due to its ability to conduct electrical currents, shungite is a wonderful tool in Reiki work. Use shungite on the body wherever you would like to increase or direct the flow of energy.

Angels & Deities

Shungite has a connection with Mars, the ancient Roman god of war and a supreme protector.

As a Pairing

Shungite and **SELENITE** create a beautiful balance of energy: pure, uplifting light and the protection that lies in shadow. Shungite works well with other grounding stones such as **HEMATITE** too. It combines beautifully with the fiery energy of **RUBY**, each enhancing the power of the other, as happens to a degree with shungite and other stones due to its conductive nature. Pair with **BLACK ONYX** for exponentially increased protective energies.

HEALING PROPERTIES

Mental & Emotional

Shungite is very effective for ridding yourself of toxic emotions, stress, anxiety, or negative thought patterns. The nickname of the "miracle stone" doesn't seem far-fetched once you've experienced its profoundly detoxifying effects. It is also extremely grounding, helping you move through your days with more ease and stability.

Spiritual

There may be no more potent cleanser of the auric field than this lustrous mineral. Not only will it remove electromagnetic frequencies and unwanted energies from your personal space, but it will also work to remove you from toxic people and situations. Shungite conducts energy and amplifies the effects of other stones.

Physical

Shungite has been used to purify water for centuries in Russia—the Russian tsar Peter the Great was well aware of its properties and established a healing spa near the original deposit in Shunga village. It supports the immune system and is said to be anti-inflammatory. Its effects on free radicals and cell damage have been studied for years.

SELENITE

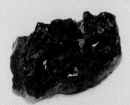

RUBY

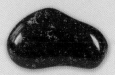

BLACK ONYX

FOR YOUR STAR SIGN

Shungite can be a useful tool for those who are born under the sign of Cancer. Cancerians are highly sensitive and emotionally intuitive—frequently finding themselves drained and running on empty as a result. Often, those born under the sign of the crab need to retreat into their shell, and shungite can be used to fortify boundaries and protect their energy. Its purifying qualities are also incredibly valuable, ridding the aura of any draining energy that may be lingering.

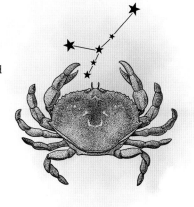

BLACK ONYX

"THE STONE OF PROTECTION"

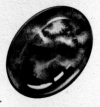

APPEARANCE

Onyx is a layered form of chalcedony, which is a type of microcrystalline quartz. It can have black and white bands of color, or appear as solid black. With true onyx, you will see a waxy luster on the surface, although it can also be polished to look glossy.

MEANING

The most ancient and revered black stone, onyx has no rival when it comes to providing protection against negative energy. The name onyx is derived from the Greek word for "fingernail" or "claw."

RARITY

Natural black onyx that has not been treated is on the rarer side, but not unobtainable. Be wary of buying black glass or dyed chalcedony.

HEALING PROPERTIES

Mental & Emotional

Black onyx supports emotional strength and stability, and also encourages confident decision-making. This stone can help you to move through the stages of grief and other emotional traumas. It keeps the energy around you calm and dispels any negativity that may leave you feeling drained, exhausted, or discouraged.

Spiritual

Black onyx literally shields the aura from any negative or toxic energy. It keeps you grounded and protected, especially during any type of psychic or meditative work. It can be helpful when working through past-life issues or trauma, as well as for identifying karmic patterns in your life.

Physical

Black onyx can be used to support physical vitality on so many levels. If you're feeling sluggish, lethargic, or bloated, carry a piece in your pocket. As black onyx is a root chakra stone, it can assist with problems in the feet, legs, and lower back. It can also be supportive for the reproductive organs and digestive system.

IN A DAILY RITUAL

Throughout history, humans have ritualized the wearing of onyx. Ancient Roman soldiers would wear it into battle for protection, while legend states that even Cleopatra wore it to keep herself safe from harm. Wear a piece of onyx, preferably against the skin, if you find yourself heading into situations that may feel dangerous or are energetically draining.

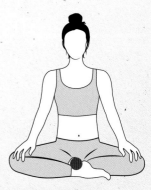

WORKING WITH THE CHAKRAS

Black onyx speaks directly to muladhara, the root chakra. This chakra keeps us grounded into the earth and is responsible for releasing any negativity we may be holding. It is crucial to keep this energy center unblocked and balanced, or we may suffer in all other areas of our lives; our most basic feelings of security and safety depend on this. It is of particular importance when embarking on any spiritual work. Black onyx speaks to us of balance, duality, yin and yang; it beseeches us to expand spiritually while keeping us safe and grounded through muladhara.

IN A CRYSTAL GRID

Use the "Flower of Life" grid for this crystal (see page 122). Often, when we are called to work with crystals, it is because we are highly sensitive people, vulnerable to the energies around us and with innate gifts of intuition and telepathic abilities that the world needs. If you identify as an empath or highly sensitive person, consider using this grid to safeguard your soft heart. Use clear quartz in the center as the focus stone. Add pearls in the way stone position—these are symbolic of your inner gifts and the need for a hard, outer shell at times. Enter powerful black onyx in the desire stone position.

FOR YOUR STAR SIGN

Black onyx is the perfect counterpart for those born under the sign of Leo. Leo's personality is exuberant and infectious, but can sometimes benefit from tempering. Carrying this ancient talisman provides Leos with the grounding, calming, and balance that can really benefit the sign. The intensity of this fire sign can also lead to burnout, making onyx's ability to replenish and recharge very useful.

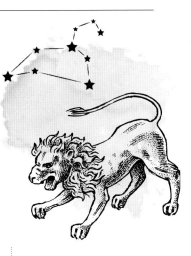

For Protection

Whether by safeguarding soldiers in battle, travelers on voyages, or mystics contacting other realms, this ancient stone is synonymous with protection. Onyx dissipates negative energy instantly, keeping your energy field clear. Since ancient times, it has been used to ward off evil spirits, impart strength, and bring good fortune.

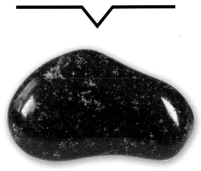

Black onyx

Angels & Deities

It is said that when Cupid cut his mother Venus's fingernails, they floated to the bottom of the Indus River and became the white bands in the black stones.

—— In Reiki ——

Black onyx's association with the root chakra means it can be used to balance any area in the body's lower half. Healers should carry a piece of onyx on their body to safeguard them against picking up negative energy.

& As a Pairing

Black onyx is compatible with nearly all stones, serving as an energetic bodyguard while they do their work. It matches well with light-colored stones like **WHITE HOWLITE** or **PEARL**, and balances the pure white light of **SELENITE** beautifully. Anyone embarking on deep, spiritual work can also pair black onyx with **LAPIS LAZULI**. Try combining black onyx with **SHUNGITE** for exponentially increased energies of protection.

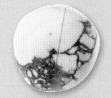

WHITE HOWLITE

PEARL

LAPIS LAZULI

HEMATITE

"THE STONE OF THE MIND"

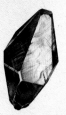

APPEARANCE
HEMATITE crystal has a metallic luster and is usually silvery black in color, but can also be seen in tones of brown or red. It is iron oxide–based, and one of the most common minerals on the planet.

MEANING
The name hematite is derived from the Greek word for "blood" due to its high iron content. Hematite is known for having strong properties of protection, grounding, and strength.

RARITY
Luckily for us, hematite is generally quite affordable and abundant. The largest production site of hematite in the world is in the Lake Superior district in North America.

HEALING PROPERTIES

Mental & Emotional
Hematite is wonderful for promoting mental clarity, memory, focus, and concentration. It grounds and protects us, being especially useful for empaths and highly sensitive people. Hematite can help move us out of a negative emotional spiral toward more logic-based thinking and problem-solving.

Spiritual
Hematite is a great ally when deepening your spiritual practice, as its grounding energies will keep you tethered to this realm. Meditating with hematite can yield profound results, as new heights can only be reached when the roots are firmly planted. Hematite can increase your overall sense of harmony in life.

Physical
Due to its high iron content, hematite has been used historically for issues of the blood—for example, it would be carried onto the battlefield or laid by the bedside during childbirth. To this day, it can be used for detoxification, circulatory issues, high blood pressure, or problems with menstruation.

For Protection

Hematite is one of the most protective stones on the planet, and humans have intuited this since ancient times. It can absorb negative energy like a sponge, so make sure to cleanse your hematite stone often! Wearing hematite throughout the day keeps you safe, centered, and energized.

IN A DAILY RITUAL
One of the simplest and most accessible ways to harness the power of a crystal's energy on a daily basis is by wearing it, and there's no shortage of affordable hematite beads and jewelry. When you're feeling scatterbrained, sluggish, or as if your head is up in the clouds, try wearing a bracelet of hematite or carry a tumbled stone in your pocket throughout the day.

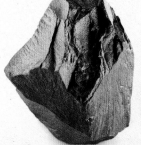
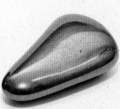

Hematite

IN A CRYSTAL GRID

Use the "Metatron's Cube" grid for this crystal (see page 123). Hematite is an exciting stone to include in grid work due to its strong energy flow and protective qualities. It infuses any crystal arrangement with a vital life-force energy that supercharges all other elements. If you're seeking to deepen your spiritual practice, combine hematite with clear quartz for a road map to guide and protect you on your path. Place hematite in the way stone position and surround with more clear quartz as the desire stones. This will protect you with earth energy and keep you grounded as you venture further toward spiritual awakening.

FOR YOUR STAR SIGN

Hematite can be a wonderful match for the signs of Aries and Aquarius. Fiery, impulsive Aries may benefit from hematite's cooling clarity. The grounding energy of this metallic stone helps to balance the Aries ram. Aquarians, on the other hand, can sometimes take on too much of the energy around them, making hematite a valuable tool for them for emotional protection. It can assist the water-bearer in manifesting some of those wild dreams that Aquarians are known for, but often lack the follow-through required to achieve.

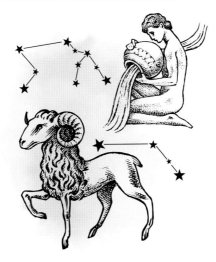

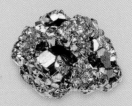

&

As a Pairing

Pair hematite with **PYRITE** for a compatible yet subtle play of energies; each amplifies the vibrations of the other. Hematite works well with all other grounding stones such as **BLACK TOURMALINE** and **SHUNGITE**. For a wonderful balance of energies, combine with **CLEAR QUARTZ**—the heaviness of hematite is uplifted by the light, soaring energy of clear quartz. Use hematite to bring grounding balance to **TOPAZ'S** fiery mood.

PYRITE

BLACK TOURMALINE

SHUNGITE

——— In Reiki ———

Hematite is very effective in lower chakra energy healing. Place on or around the root and sacral chakras to bring balance, restoration, and grounding to these vital energy centers.

Angels & Deities

Hematite is associated with Mars, the Roman god of war.

WORKING WITH THE CHAKRAS

Muladhara, the root chakra, is where you'll feel the pull of this amazing mineral. Hematite is so ever-present in the earth's crust, it is no wonder that it has such a strong, grounding earth energy. Wearing or working with hematite literally connects us to the earth beneath, specifically through muladhara. This chakra governs feelings of safety and security; when it is blocked or imbalanced, you may struggle with excessive fear, anxiety, or depression. Let hematite be a tether and reminder that you are a perfect part of this earth: strong, connected, and powerful.

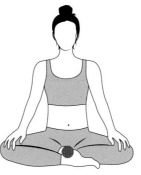

TIGER'S EYE

"THE STONE OF STRENGTH"

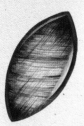

APPEARANCE

TIGER'S EYE is a chatoyant mineral, most often occurring with bands of brown and gold, but also found in red and blue hues. It is a member of the chalcedony family of minerals, and resembles the eye of a cat—powerful, mysterious, and bewitching.

MEANING

Tiger's eye is an ancient symbol of protection and inner strength. It emboldens the lower chakras—the solar plexus, sacral, and root chakras—bringing us renewed confidence, clarity, and willpower.

RARITY

Tiger's eye is both accessible and abundant (the chief source being South Africa), which makes it an easy addition to a crystal toolkit.

FOR YOUR STAR SIGN

Those born under Gemini will have a kinship with this special stone. Tiger's eye is a crystal of duality and harmony, with light glinting off threads of quartz and tiny shadows and dark valleys producing an optical display—light and dark, overt brilliance and subtlety. Geminians thrive in this energy of balance. Tiger's eye represents both the earth and the sun, giving grounding and nourishing energy to the often-scattered Gemini.

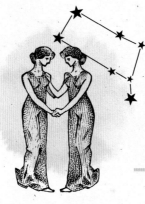

Angels & Deities

Tiger's eye claims connection with the Egyptian deities of Ra, god of the sun, and Bastet, the goddess of protection.

IN A CRYSTAL GRID

Use the "Metatron's Cube" grid for this crystal (see page 123). Tiger's eye performs wonderfully in crystal grid work in the way stone position, connecting the inner and outer crystals. This is because way stones provide a "way" for your intention to be manifested and tiger's eye is known as a stone of action and energy. So, create a grid for manifestation and accomplishing a goal, using a citrine crystal as the focus stone and pyrite pieces as desire stones. This formula symbolizes that your intention is to create an energy of abundance by taking appropriate action.

For Protection

Many ancient civilizations attributed qualities of protection and good fortune to this powerful stone. Roman soldiers would wear it into battle. Ancient Egyptians, Chinese, and Greeks—to name a few—all considered it a talisman of protection and good fortune, some even believing it would ward off the evil eye and spirits.

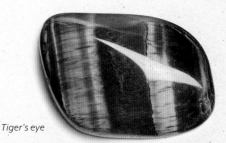

Tiger's eye

In Reiki

In Reiki healing, tiger's eye is usually placed over the root chakra or solar plexus chakra, depending on where there seems to be an imbalance. You can also charge a crystal and carry it with you through the day.

WORKING WITH THE CHAKRAS

This gem resonates with the lower chakras, but particularly with manipura, the solar plexus chakra. The Sanskrit *manipura* roughly translates as "city of jewels," meaning this chakra is a center of personal light, resplendence, and possibility. When you're open and allow energy to flow freely, you begin to see self-imposed limitations lift away. Tiger's eye and its primitive energy invites us to own our inner strength and potential. Your "city of jewels" is before you: a landscape dotted with your wildest dreams that you finally have the courage to grasp.

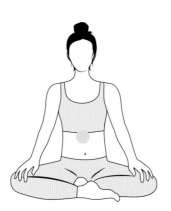

HEALING PROPERTIES

Mental & Emotional

Tiger's eye has an empowering, energizing effect on our emotional state. It helps us to realize our inner strength and potential, and then the courage to share that with the world. Assertiveness can often be mistaken for aggression or egocentrism, but this crystal ally helps us to be bold yet graceful.

Spiritual

Tiger's eye sends energy to the lower chakras, grounding us and keeping us tethered while we explore our spirituality. It brings harmony to our lives, as well as a deep sense of comfort and an acceptance of where we find ourselves in the present moment. It helps us to realize our karma in this life.

Physical

If you feel sluggish, unmotivated, or run-down, tiger's eye is a good antidote. It awakens life-force energy (*chi* in Chinese and *prana* in Sanskrit) and assists with a struggling metabolism or sex drive. Tiger's eye can be cleansing to the blood and the endocrine system.

IN A DAILY RITUAL

Use the energy of the sun to really tap into the strength and message of tiger's eye. Allow the stone to sit in direct sunlight for several hours, then find a comfortable seat and hold it in your right hand. Feel the warmth of the sun spreading from your hand to all the cells of your body. This is a lovely exercise to carry into the colder winter months, when seasonal depression creeps in for many.

& As a Pairing

CITRINE and tiger's eye are perfect companions. The strength provided by tiger's eye catapults us into citrine's energy of abundance and prosperity. Additionally, combining tiger's eye with **PYRITE** creates a forceful duo. The energy of the sun and earth combine, and the result is a brew that leaves you energized and standing tall in your power. Great magic can also occur if you pair tiger's eye with **LABRADORITE**. If working with **MOLDAVITE** and its lessons feel too intense, then pair with tiger's eye for courage of the heart.

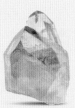

CITRINE

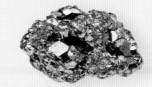

PYRITE

SMOKY QUARTZ

"THE STONE OF GROUNDING"

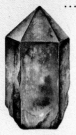

APPEARANCE

SMOKY QUARTZ is a variety of quartz crystal, ranging from a light, champagne color to a dark chocolate-brown. The color is a product of natural radiation in the earth. Most often available in crystal clusters or points, tumbled stones, faceted gems, and carvings.

MEANING

Smoky quartz is more or less synonymous with grounding, earthly connection, protection from negative energies, and transmutation of those energies to positive ones.

RARITY

Luckily for us, smoky quartz is widely available and makes an easy (and recommended) addition to any crystal collection.

HEALING PROPERTIES

Mental & Emotional

Smoky quartz is an invaluable tool for anyone who often finds themselves "scatterbrained" or who struggles to be fully present or grounded. This form of quartz maintains a strong, energetic connection to the earth, and so when we carry or work with it, we find ourselves more tethered, grounded, and focused.

Spiritual

This invaluable stone literally turns negative energy to positive, surrounding us with an aura of protection and purification. This raising of our energy level puts us into a higher state of consciousness. As we remain rooted in deep earth energy, we feel safe and free to let go of what no longer serves us.

Physical

Smoky quartz is a friend to the digestive system, and facilitates the absorption of beneficial minerals. It may also provide protection from radiation and electromagnetic smog.

IN A DAILY RITUAL

For a daily practice in grounding and connecting to the earth, first find a comfortable seat in a chair. Rest a smoky quartz beneath your feet, positioning it gently so as not to damage the crystal. Visualize energy flowing up from the earth into your feet, filling your body with the sweet, humming energy from the earth below. If you find yourself getting stressed throughout the day, refer back to this mental image and feel your constant earthly connection.

WORKING WITH THE CHAKRAS

Muladhara—the first or root chakra, located at the base of the spine—is perfectly matched to smoky quartz's grounding vibrations. Although it is a darker, "lower chakra" crystal, some forms of smoky quartz will create an energetic connection all the way up through the crown chakra, awakening *kundalini* energy. The root chakra connects us to the earth, our physical bodies, basic primitive needs and instincts, and our ancestors, making its proper function a necessity for anyone seeking grounding or a sense of stability in the world.

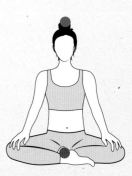

IN A CRYSTAL GRID

Use the "Square" grid for this crystal (see page 123). Smoky quartz is perfect for adding an element of protection to any grid. Whether the intention is guarding the home, family, or heart, this stone is invaluable. It is ideal for a grid to safeguard an open heart, perhaps when embarking on a romantic relationship or navigating troubles in an existing one. Use smoky quartz as the focus stone, rose quartz crystals as the way stone, and malachite as the desire stones.

FOR YOUR STAR SIGN

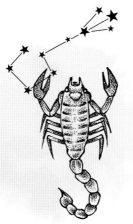

Those born under the sign of Scorpio will find a well-suited companion in smoky quartz. Scorpios tend toward darkness and secrecy, as this astrological phase marks our transition to the darker, colder seasons. Smoky quartz helps to ground that brooding, intense energy, allowing Scorpios access to their own inner truth and clarity. It can also help this star sign to access their innate psychic ability.

For Protection

One of the premier stones for protecting the aura, smoky quartz is a good candidate to work with in jewelry form, and the piece can be worn every day. It envelops the wearer in the supportive energy of the earth, gently detoxifying and shielding him or her.

—— In Reiki ——

Place a large smoky quartz cluster at your feet or on the root chakra during a healing session. Alternatively, you can put one cluster underneath the table in order to ground and purify the whole session.

Angels & Deities

Smoky quartz was sacred to the ancient Druids. It was also associated with Hecate, the Greek goddess of witchcraft and the occult.

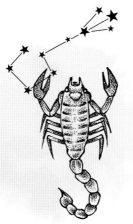

Smoky quartz

& As a Pairing

Try pairing smoky quartz with **MALACHITE**, so the heart is open, but protected from negative energy. Smoky quartz and **BLACK TOURMALINE** also make a powerful protective pairing, while combining it with any form of quartz, such as **CLEAR QUARTZ**, is always effective. For root chakra healing, pair smoky quartz with dark-colored or red stones like **RED CORAL**. The grounding energy of smoky quartz can be used to create safe boundaries when working with the heart-healing energy of **EMERALD**.

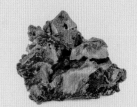

MALACHITE

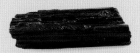

BLACK TOURMALINE

DRAVITE

"THE STONE FOR WOUNDED HEARTS"

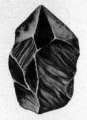

APPEARANCE

DRAVITE is a light to dark brown member of the tourmaline family, ranging from near-translucent to opaque. It is occasionally faceted, but mostly found in its raw form. When dravite is dark in color, it can be mistaken for black tourmaline.

MEANING

Dravite, which is also known as champagne tourmaline, was named for the site of its discovery—the Drava River in Slovenia. It is known for its grounding connection to the earth and also for its detoxifying and protective abilities.

RARITY

Although a very common mineral, dravite falls into the category of lesser-known crystals for healing. Large crystals and rare transparent forms command higher prices.

WORKING WITH THE CHAKRAS

Dravite is predominantly a root chakra stone, but what makes it unique as a grounding crystal is that it connects with the heart chakra as well. This dualistic nature makes the brown-colored tourmaline a rare gem in the realm of crystal healing. The more balanced our root chakra (muladhara) becomes, the safer we feel and the more we allow our heart chakra (anahata) to open and receive love. This signifies a necessary connection between the two energy centers, one that is often overlooked when working with only one or the other.

For Protection

Dravite is an incredibly effective protector of the energetic body. It shields us from psychic attack, making it a perfect stone to carry if you work in a busy, draining environment. Its connection to the earth will help to transmute all negative energy to positive as it enters your aura.

IN A DAILY RITUAL

If you're finding yourself feeling scattered, drained, or lethargic, try this simple ritual to bring some regenerative and grounding energy into your life. Take a piece of dravite and bury it outside in the soil for twenty-four hours.

This supercharges the dravite with healing earth energy. Carry the stone with you throughout the day and hold it in your (nondominant, receiving) hand whenever you face moments of heightened stress.

Angels & Deities

Although not associated with any specific deity, dravite can be used to connect with Mother Earth or any of the spirits of nature.

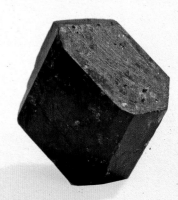

Dravite

FOR YOUR STAR SIGN

Dravite tourmaline makes a wonderful crystal companion for those born in the first sign of the zodiac, Aries. The sign of the ram is driven, motivated, and magnetic. All of that fire sign energy may get a lot accomplished, but can also lead quickly to burnout. Use dravite to bring in some much-needed balance and temperance. It can help to quell a quick temper and bring a sense of perspective to frenzied situations.

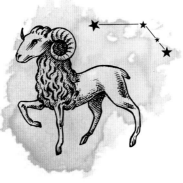

HEALING PROPERTIES

Mental & Emotional
Most members of the tourmaline family carry a soothing, detoxifying, and regenerative energy, and dravite is no exception. It is particularly useful for balancing the left and right hemispheres of the brain, and encourages emotional equilibrium, allowing you to release old trauma with compassion and strength.

Spiritual
Typical of dark-colored, grounding stones, dravite assists with spiritual work by maintaining an energetic tether to the earthly plane. While meditating or exploring our higher chakras, brown tourmaline ensures we are protected from negative energy. Its connection to the earth enhances our spiritual connection with Mother Nature.

Physical
Dravite provides constant detoxification of the body and helps with the removal of blockages. It can also help to regenerate stressed or ailing organs, including the skin. The lymphatic system, circulatory system, and intestines can all benefit from daily wearing or working with this warm, cola-colored crystal.

IN A CRYSTAL GRID

Use the "Square" grid for this crystal (see page 123). The perfect grid for dravite tourmaline is one designed to protect and fortify the heart. This can be useful when dealing with relationship issues: either beginning or ending one, or navigating through a tough period. A square-shaped grid is ideal for this due to its inherent protective energy. Rose quartz or green garnet make a perfect focus stone. Surround this with dravite, black tourmaline, or any strong, protective crystals that you are drawn to. When dealing with the heart, adding a personal element is very effective: a photograph, keepsake, written mantra, or anything that feels poignant for you.

—————— In Reiki ——————

Use dravite tourmaline as a tool in energy work to connect the root and heart chakras. Literally draw a line between these two centers and visualize a string of energy running between them.

As a Pairing

Pair dravite with **TSAVORITE**, which is also known as green garnet, for the ultimate cocktail of rejuvenating, heart-healing energy. Additionally, experiment by combining dravite with other grounding stones for amplified energies—**BLACK TOURMALINE** in particular makes a great combination. All colors of tourmaline can be paired for different energetic outcomes.

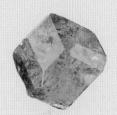

TSAVORITE

BLACK TOURMALINE

CLEAR QUARTZ

"THE MASTER HEALER"

APPEARANCE

CLEAR QUARTZ is one of the most recognizable and renowned members of the mineral kingdom. It is transparent, colorless, and varies widely in formation, but is usually seen in clusters or single terminations.

MEANING

Quartz crystal (also known as rock crystal) is known for its ability to absorb, store, and amplify energy. Its myriad uses in the fields of science, technology, metaphysics, and healing are testament to its power and versatility.

RARITY

Luckily for us, quartz is one of the most common and abundant minerals on earth, which means it is easily acquired by crystal collectors.

HEALING PROPERTIES

Mental & Emotional

Clear quartz is referred to as the "master healer" for good reason. It can be used to amplify all positive energy and also to cleanse the aura of negativity, toxicity, and fear. The enlightening effects of clear quartz provide increased mental clarity, insight, and emotional stability.

Spiritual

Clear quartz is a special gift from the earth to further us along our spiritual path and align us with our highest selves. This stone is unique in that it can be programmed with a specific energy or intention, which makes it an invaluable tool for meditation, visualization, and manifestation.

Physical

Clear quartz strengthens the immune system, bolstering our resistance to disease and imbalance. It also boosts the metabolism and helps the body to absorb nutrients and rid itself of toxins. Clear quartz can also be useful in treating migraines, vertigo, and motion sickness.

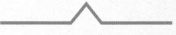

Clear quartz

IN A DAILY RITUAL

You can use clear quartz to recharge other crystals and stones. Clear quartz is piezoelectric, meaning it can convert energy of one kind into another. This is what makes its technological applications so vast and allows it to cleanse other crystals of any negative energy. Quartz clusters, geodes, slabs, and large points work well for this purpose—simply place your other stone on top and leave overnight.

For Protection

Clear quartz crystal has been recognized as one of the most protective stones by various civilizations since the beginning of time, being used for many things, from safeguarding soldiers to guiding the souls of the dead. In modern days, in addition to shielding the aura, it is believed to protect against EMF frequencies and radiation.

FOR YOUR STAR SIGN

Clear quartz, along with diamond, is the birthstone for the month of April, and is auspicious for both Aries and Taurus. These are the signs that begin the cycle of the zodiac, and arrive with vigor and passionate energy—too much, at times, which can lead to burnout and exhaustion for the signs of the ram and the bull. Clear quartz can provide much-needed tempering and calming, encouraging patience and a sense of balance.

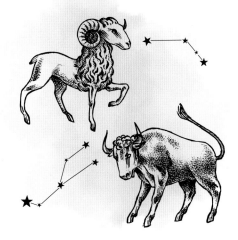

—— In Reiki ——

Clear quartz is one of the most commonly used tools in Reiki healing. Use quartz points as wands to direct energy throughout the body, clear blockages, or intensify the effects of other stones.

Angels & Deities

Clear quartz is connected to Kundalini, who is the Hindu goddess of life-force energy.

IN A CRYSTAL GRID

Use the "Tripod of Life" grid for this crystal (see page 123). The power and versatility of clear quartz cannot be overstated; it can be used in nearly any kind of crystal grid. It is most commonly used as the focus stone due to its ability to draw universal energy and transmit it throughout the grid. For an easy, unique, and potent grid, try composing one entirely of clear quartz. Following the Tripod of Life grid pattern, arrange quartz pieces in the focus, way, and desire stone positions as you see fit. Set your intention clearly and carefully, as the quartz is "programmable" by your thoughts and vibration.

WORKING WITH THE CHAKRAS

Clear quartz can be used to open and align all of the chakras, but is specifically linked with the crown chakra located at the top of the head. The Sanskrit name for this chakra is *sahasrara*, and it is the center of our spiritual connection. Due to this crystal's ability to absorb and transmit energetic vibrations, simply having a piece of clear quartz anywhere in your space will positively impact chakric function. For deeper work, try meditating with clear quartz and visualize that energy center above the head opening up like a lotus blossom (*sahasrara* translates to "thousand-petaled").

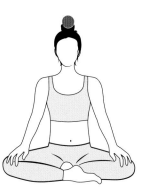

& As a Pairing

Clear quartz is almost universally compatible with other crystals and stones, but resonates most strongly with other members of the quartz family, namely **SMOKY QUARTZ**, **ROSE QUARTZ**, and **CITRINE**. Clear quartz will always amplify energy, so keep that in mind when creating crystal pairings, particularly if you are using stones with a high vibration.

SMOKY QUARTZ

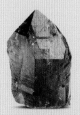

ROSE QUARTZ

CITRINE

MOONSTONE

"THE TRAVELER'S STONE"

APPEARANCE

MOONSTONE is in the feldspar family of minerals. It glows with a shimmer known as adularescence. Although it's most commonly seen in milky white or "rainbow," it can also be found in colors such as peach, blue, green, brown, gray, and black.

MEANING

Since ancient times, the beautiful moonstone has been treasured and sought after due to its mystical connection with the moon, both in terms of its physical resemblance and its gentle, feminine energy.

RARITY

Moonstones range greatly in appearance and also value, from a very affordable pocket stone to a beautiful piece of fine jewelry.

WORKING WITH THE CHAKRAS

The third eye and crown chakras both benefit from working with moonstone crystal. Telepathic, clairvoyant abilities are heightened when working with moonstone—for optimal effect, place the stone between your eyebrows during meditation. This will expand your inherent powers of intuition. The crown chakra, our center of spiritual awakening, also responds beautifully to working with this stone. Moonstone emits a white light, wrapping us in protective energies and encouraging us to grow through spiritual expansion. Keeping the pathway open between these two chakras is the key to achieving spiritual growth and healing.

IN A DAILY RITUAL

Harness moonstone's power to connect to the dreamworld by placing a stone underneath your pillow at night. Bonus points for charging in the moonlight first! This simple ritual will encourage lucid dreaming and also facilitate dream recall. Make sure to keep a journal beside your bed to capture your memories first thing in the morning.

In Reiki

Use moonstone for any energy work centered around feminine issues. It is often used to enhance fertility or regulate menstrual cycles. Any color of moonstone will suffice, but white and peach are particularly effective for this work.

For Protection

Moonstone is protective both psychically and energetically. It creates a shield of light around the aura, connecting you with fierce, goddess energy. It was known as the "traveler's stone," since it protected travelers at night, lighting their path to safety.

Moonstone

HEALING PROPERTIES

Mental & Emotional
Moonstone brings with it balance and fluidity. This beautiful stone imparts a feminine, calming energy and can also be used to bring a sense of perspective to troubling situations. It can help calm us down and reduce feelings of tension. Moonstone reminds us that there is a season and a cycle for everything.

Spiritual
Goddess energy abounds with the glimmering moonstone! Powerful, sensual, and healing, use this crystal to connect with divine feminine energy and your own powers of intuition. Moonstone adds a touch of magic to the everyday. It can also be very helpful with dreamwork.

Physical
Moonstone is a special friend to women. With its connection to the cycles of nature, moonstone makes a great companion for anyone who is suffering from PMS or infertility, for example, or with other issues of the reproductive system. It can also help ease the pain felt during menstruation or even childbirth.

Angels & Deities

Moonstone was connected to the Roman moon goddess Diana, and thought to bring love and good fortune to the wearer. It was also considered sacred in the Hindu faith, linked with the god Ganesh.

IN A CRYSTAL GRID
Use the "Seed of Life" grid for this crystal (see page 122), ideally during a full moon for potency, using moonstone to honor your inner goddess (both men and women can benefit from honoring the divine feminine). Use kunzite as the focus stone, amethyst as the way stone, and moonstone as the desire stones. Can you feel the strong, sweet, feminine energy radiating? Intuitively accent with organic materials: lilac blossom, rose petals, or red clover are perfect.

FOR YOUR STAR SIGN
Moonstone is a birthstone for the month of June, and so aligns with the sign of Gemini. This is the first air sign of the zodiac year, and so moonstone hangs perfectly in its space. Geminians show such excitement about, and curiosity for, the world around them that they can sometimes become overwhelmed by it all. Moonstone makes a perfect touchstone for this star sign, keeping Geminians calm, centered, and attuned to their own needs.

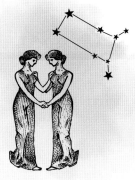

& As a Pairing

Pair moonstone with its astral twin, **SUNSTONE**, for a balancing effect on your aura. These crystals work as yin and yang to keep you in check emotionally and energetically. Another beloved companion is **LABRADORITE**, which compounds the mystical effects of moonstone. Try amplifying **PEARL'S** moon connection in grids or rituals by pairing it with moonstone. Pairing with **KUNZITE** also enhances moonstone's divine feminine energies.

SUNSTONE

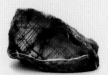

LABRADORITE

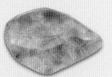

KUNZITE

HERKIMER DIAMOND

"THE STONE OF CONNECTION"

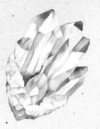

APPEARANCE

HERKIMER DIAMOND is a form of quartz crystal that naturally forms one termination at each end. True herkimer diamonds are only found in one area of New York State and are over 500 million years old. They can be smoky or perfectly clear, or contain inclusions.

MEANING

These unique gems symbolize connection: between us and spirit, between two individuals, and between the chakras. It is a truly transformative crystal for mind, body, and spirit.

RARITY

There are many double-terminated crystals sold as "herkimers," but to be assured of their authenticity, ensure you source them from the Herkimer region of New York State.

HEALING PROPERTIES

Mental & Emotional

Herkimer diamonds carry a spiritual vibration that calms a worried or anxious mind. Their presence in our energy field works to keep us balanced and in the state of mind that everything is exactly as it should be. It is said that two friends or lovers, upon parting, should each take a herkimer diamond to remain vibrationally connected.

Spiritual

Herkimers are said to have the highest vibrations of any form of quartz, with powerful manifesting and amplifying energies. They keep us connected to our highest selves, divine energy, and spirit guides/angels. They connect powerfully to the dreamworld and may be used for past-life work or astral travel.

Physical

Herkimer diamonds are purifying and can help to rid the body of unwanted toxins. They can also be used to boost a sluggish immune system or to help with low energy levels. Herkimers may also be helpful for problems with eyesight and vision, as well as chronic migraine headaches.

—— In Reiki ——

Herkimers are incredible tools for Reiki work and body layouts. Use anywhere you're seeking to amplify energy—they are particularly useful for opening chakric systems and reestablishing a free flow of energy.

IN A CRYSTAL GRID

Use the "Vesica Piscis" grid for this crystal (see page 122). Herkimers may be among the most effective stones for crystal grid work due to their shape—the double terminations allow a strong flow of energy and amplify whatever passes through. For this reason, herkimers make perfect way stones for a grid, placed between the center stone and the outer stones. If you would like to step up your spiritual work, then try creating this grid for an increased connection with spirit guides, divine energy, and crown chakra opening. Use a large cluster of clear quartz as the focus stone, herkimers as the way stones, and then phenacite as the desire stones.

IN A DAILY RITUAL

Herkimer diamonds hold a special connection to the dreamworld. Utilize their power of connecting us to other realms by placing one under your pillow at night. Keeping a dream journal by your bedside is also helpful. Herkimer diamonds can enhance lucid dreaming, as well as dream recall. Before going to sleep, hold the herkimer diamond and ask it to show you what it would like you to see.

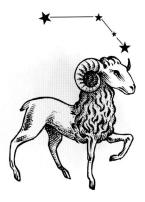

FOR YOUR STAR SIGN

As an alternative birthstone for the month of April, herkimer diamonds have a special connection with those who are born under the sign of Aries, as both are ruled by the planet Mars. The first sign of the zodiacal year, the star sign Aries symbolizes freshness and purity of spirit. Aries wants to blaze new trails, bring in fresh ideas, and create an adventure-filled life. Call upon herkimer diamond if you wish to connect with your highest potential and calling!

WORKING WITH THE CHAKRAS

The crown chakra connects beautifully with the herkimer diamond. The Sanskrit term for this chakra (which is located at the top of the head) is *sahasrara*. This translates as "thousand-petaled," in reference to the thousand-petaled lotus blossom that is said to represent this energetic doorway to the divine. The herkimer is considered one of the most effective openers for sahasrara, and makes a perfect meditation tool for this reason. Due to their ability to facilitate the flow of energy, however, herkimers can help open any chakra that may be blocked.

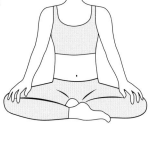

For Protection

The herkimer diamond is highly protective. It shields the aura with a pure, healing light and can even be used to protect spaces, either by creating a room grid or a crystal elixir for spraying. It is also useful if you want to protect yourself from electromagnetic frequencies.

Angels & Deities

The Mohawk tribe of Native Americans considered herkimers to be "spirit stones" and held them sacred as a result, using them in jewelry, rituals, and burials.

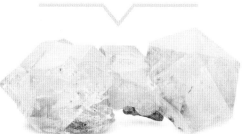

Herkimer diamond

& As a Pairing

As with most forms of quartz, the herkimer diamond pairs with almost any stone. Although it brings out the fullest energetic potential of any crystal, it vibrates particularly well with high-vibration stones such as **SERAPHINITE** and **PHENACITE**. It can bring much-needed grounding energy when paired with ethereal **K2 JASPER**. To enhance the herkimer diamond's crown chakra connection, try pairing it with **MOLDAVITE**.

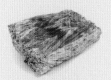

SERAPHINITE

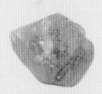

PHENACITE

K2 JASPER

PEARL

"THE GEMSTONE OF DIVINE WISDOM"

APPEARANCE

PEARL, one of the oldest and most treasured adornments on the planet, is a combination of mineral and organic material, formed within the living tissue of a mollusk. It can be found in an array of colors, and exhibits a natural iridescence known as "pearlescence."

MEANING

Pearl falls into the category of "organic gemstone" in the same way as red coral or amber. Highly prized for millennia, pearl has come to symbolize prestige, purity, wisdom, and introspection.

RARITY

Natural pearls are quite rare and valuable, and so cultured pearls were developed in Asia in the 1800s to make this beautiful "stone" more affordable.

WORKING WITH THE CHAKRAS

Pearl is a stone of higher wisdom and intuition, and while it works well with several points of energy along the body, it is best paired with the crown chakra. Sahasrara, our seventh and highest major chakra, located at the top of the head, is the source of our spiritual connection. This chakra connects us to our own innate wisdom as well as the higher consciousness of the universe—when it is free of blockages and allows the unhindered flow of energy. Let the soothing energy of pearl caress your crown chakra into a state of gentle, spiritual balance.

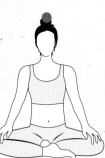

IN A DAILY RITUAL

The illustrious pearl, with all its beauty and mythology, is the result of one tiny irritant in the shell of a mollusk and nature's ability to nurture, protect, and heal itself. Meditate with pearl when working through trauma, inner child healing, or anything in your life that seems to have embedded in your consciousness. Draw on pearl's divine wisdom, adaptability, and protective energies to guard and guide you.

Angels & Deities

Indian mythology connects pearls with the god Krishna, who plucked the first one from the ocean for his daughter's wedding jewelry.

— In Reiki —

Use pearl on the body anywhere there is heat or imbalance. Utilize pearl's stabilizing, calming effects for energy work and wear it as a healer to remain protected, balanced, and intuitively connected.

For Protection

Pearl is said to absorb the negative energy of the wearer and transmute it to a more beautiful, light-filled vibration. It is also said to protect lovers, making it a popular wedding gift. Children are also protected by pearl, which is why a piece of pearl jewelry is such a great choice for little ones.

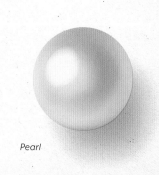

Pearl

IN A CRYSTAL GRID

Use the "Metatron's Cube" grid for this crystal (see page 123), with pearl to honor that feminine celestial body, the moon. This grid is perfect on full or new moon nights to connect with the regenerative energy of the lunar cycle. Put a piece of moonstone in the focus stone position. Surround with selenite wands as the way stones and pearls as the desire stones. Ideally, leave the grid outside or by a window to absorb the moonlight. Use this grid to call on your inner goddess and attune to the balance of the natural world.

HEALING PROPERTIES

Mental & Emotional
Pearl holds a deep connection to the moon and the cycles of the natural world, so turn to it for emotional balance. It holds a serene, stabilizing energy, attuning us to the natural ebb and flow of the universe. Pearl truly carries an energy of ancient wisdom and the pursuit of inner truth.

Spiritual
In Hindu, Buddhist, and Taoist traditions, the "flaming pearl" is a symbol of divine wisdom. It is said to bring cleansing, healing energy to the aura. Due to the nature of their formation, pearls are deeply associated with growth, transformation, and insightfulness. They connect with the divine feminine and goddess energy.

Physical
Pearl's connection to the moon makes it a great companion for menstruating women, helping to relieve hormonal imbalances. It can also enhance fertility and make childbirth easier. Pearls contain calcium, amino acids, magnesium, and more, making them effective in healing wounds, reducing inflammation, and aiding skin health.

FOR YOUR STAR SIGN

Pearls are the birthstone for June and the astrological gemstone for those born under the signs of Cancer and Gemini. Cancer, a water sign, makes an obvious match for this maritime gemstone. Cancer is an emotional, loyal, and sensitive sign that benefits from pearl's ability to bring comfort and protection. Gemini, the sign of the twins, also finds a match in pearl. It helps to bring balance to Gemini's duality and calm this sign's often-fiery nature.

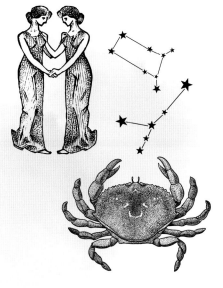

& As a Pairing

OPAL'S high water content makes it perfect with aqueous pearl. The fire of opal meets pearl's subtle iridescence in a lovely balance of energies. To amplify pearl's moon connection, combine with **MOONSTONE** or **SELENITE**. Match pearl with its nautical cousin, **RED CORAL**, for an energy of balance. Pearl also loves to be with other water element stones such as **AQUAMARINE**. It also pairs well with **BLACK ONYX**.

OPAL

MOONSTONE

SELENITE

SELENITE

"THE STONE OF PURIFICATION"

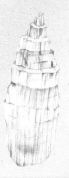

APPEARANCE

SELENITE is a translucent to whitish form of the mineral gypsum. Also known as satin spar, it forms in either flat, pane-like sheets or fibrous, silky crystallizations. Widely available in wands, carvings, and beads, it is a must-have in any crystal toolkit.

MEANING

Selenite gets its name from Selene, the Greek goddess of the moon, due to its ethereal glow that resembles moonlight. Flat sheets of selenite were once used to make windowpanes and it has, in fact, always been associated with light, purity, and protection.

RARITY

This is a very abundant mineral that should be relatively easy to acquire.

FOR YOUR STAR SIGN

Selenite connects with every astrological sign, but particularly those born under the earth sign of Taurus. Like their celestial embodiment of the bull, Taureans are strong, hardworking, and reliable. Selenite brings a lightness and gentleness to their rigid demeanor. Taureans are always pushing forward, both professionally and personally, and with selenite in hand they remain safe, protected, and clear of any toxic energies that may threaten to hold them back.

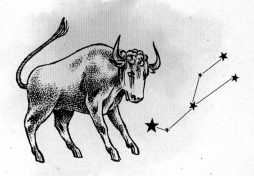

IN A DAILY RITUAL

Performing this daily ritual with a selenite wand may be one of the quickest, easiest, and most effective exercises you can use to keep yourself energetically clear and spiritually connected. Simply scan your body with the piece of selenite, holding the crystal a few inches away. Then imagine you are "brushing off" energetic debris, from head to toe.

Angels & Deities

Connects with the Greek moon goddess, Selene, who was said to pull the heavenly body across the sky in her chariot.

For Protection

This is one of the best-known stones for energetic protection. It connects to a higher realm of spirit and invokes that raised frequency to shield you from negative energy or psychic attack. In fact, it is so powerful that you can cleanse and charge your other crystals by placing them on pieces of selenite.

Selenite

WORKING WITH THE CHAKRAS

Selenite connects to the crown chakra, *sahasrara* in Sanskrit, that is located at the top of the head. This chakra symbolizes our spiritual connection and higher consciousness. A blocked crown chakra may result in anxiety or depression, feeling disconnected in life, or a desire to isolate from others. Also, anyone struggling to make a spiritual connection may have some work to do in this area. Meditating with selenite or simply keeping a piece around you in your space are both great methods for inviting its purifying light energy into your life and consciousness.

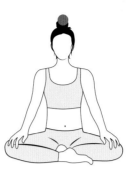

—— In Reiki ——

Perhaps one of the most useful tools for energy healing work, selenite clears the body and aura of unwanted, negative energy, as well as your physical space. Decorate with selenite liberally!

IN A CRYSTAL GRID

Use the "Square" grid for this crystal (see page 123). Selenite is such a versatile tool for grid work. Its structure means it functions like a double-terminated crystal, allowing and directing the flow of energy. It makes a great way stone for this reason, connecting separate energies, and an effective desire stone for protection grids, encircling them with pure white light. In gridding, selenite also acts as the "activator"—energetically connecting and activating all the elements at the end. To do this, take a selenite wand, hold it over the grid, and imagine connecting the crystals with an invisible line.

HEALING PROPERTIES

Mental & Emotional
Selenite is a wonderful tool for creating emotional balance. It promotes a more positive outlook in life and helps us to remain centered, even during times of stress or turmoil. The gentleness and lightness that emanates from this crystal spreads throughout our life, one feeling and situation at a time.

Spiritual
Selenite has long been associated with angelic energy, lightness, purity of spirit, and enlightenment. It is a high-vibration crystal that can be used to rid yourself of feelings of negativity. You can also use selenite to promote peace and calm. It can be used to cleanse other crystals, physical spaces, and the aura.

Physical
Selenite has intensely detoxifying effects on the physical body as well as the energetic and auric fields. It strengthens all the organs and the immune system, promotes overall good health, and has anti-aging properties. Selenite also connects very strongly with the spine and issues related to the back.

As a Pairing

Combine selenite with nearly any stone for heightened effect. High-vibration stones such as **PHENACITE** and **SERAPHINITE** pair well with selenite's soaring energies. Dark stones like **ONYX**, **BLACK TOURMALINE**, and **SHUNGITE** balance selenite's white light. Pairing selenite with **GOLDEN HEALER QUARTZ** draws in divine white light (selenite also charges this golden stone). Use selenite to amplify **PEARL'S** moon connection in grids or rituals.

PHENACITE

SERAPHINITE

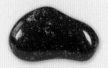

ONYX

BLACK TOURMALINE

PHENACITE

"THE ANGEL STONE"

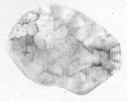

APPEARANCE

PHENACITE (or "phenakite" as it is sometimes known) presents in a range of colors, from fully transparent to white, yellow, pink, or even brown.

MEANING

The name is derived from the Greek *phenas,* which means "deceiver," as it is often mistaken for clear quartz or topaz. It is a great aid for meditation and crystal healing, but more suitable for someone experienced with crystal energy.

RARITY

Although in the rarer and pricier category, smaller, rough specimens can be found. One of the most powerful crystals, this is a highly sought-after metaphysical tool.

HEALING PROPERTIES

Mental & Emotional

Phenacite's high vibration improves mental acuity and keeps our energetic field free of negativity. Our emotions are uplifted by being close to this transformational crystal. By aligning us with the divine light and wisdom of the universe, we are able to see our problems in perspective, which lessens our worry.

Spiritual

Phenacite is one of the most effective stones for receiving messages from spiritual beings/guides, and ascended masters. It opens up avenues of divine truth and spiritual enlightenment. It can open the door to interdimensional journeying, telepathy, enhanced meditation, and dreamwork.

Physical

Providing an overall healing and purifying effect on the physical body, phenacite is particularly beneficial to brain health. Nerve damage, neurological imbalance, migraine headaches, and autoimmune disorder issues can all be eased and assisted by this powerful stone.

For Protection

Your spirit guides and guardians are constantly watching over you, and phenacite helps connect you to their vigilant energy. That "little voice" in your head, your "guardian angel," or intuition—these all stem from the same source, and phenacite plugs us into that deeply.

IN A DAILY RITUAL

When you begin working with phenacite or any high-vibration stone, start with only small increments of time and then increase these. One meditation you can practice every day is to hold a small piece of phenacite between the brows, over the third eye chakra. You may feel a warmth or slight buzzing. Begin drawing the stone upward, toward the top of your head. Imagine drawing a line between the two chakra points: the third eye and crown chakras.

Phenacite

IN A CRYSTAL GRID

Use the "Flower of Life" grid for this crystal (see page 122). Phenacite is unique in its ability to amplify the energy of other stones, which makes it a fun and effective addition to a crystal grid. A little goes a long way with this stone, so even small specimens of phenacite will pack the desired energetic punch. If you are embarking on a new (or renewed) yoga or meditation practice, create this crystal grid to achieve a "grounded" spiritual connection. To create the grid, use a piece of amethyst as the focus stone. Surround the amethyst with phenacite in the way stone position and then finish with black tourmaline as the desire stones.

FOR YOUR STAR SIGN

Those born under the sign of Gemini will find a special companion in phenacite. This special stone appeals to Gemini's intellectual curiosity. These individuals are always looking for a new horizon, adventure, or lesson… and phenacite provides this. Those with Gemini as their sign are also not afraid of transformation. The sign of the twins is ruled by the planet Mercury, which governs areas of communication, and nothing opens contact with higher, spiritual realms quite like phenacite.

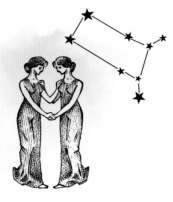

—— In Reiki ——

Phenacite is a wonderful tool for Reiki healing and any kind of crystal body layout, as it amplifies the effects of other stones in its presence. If using on its own, place between the brows or over the head to send energy into the higher chakras.

Angels & Deities

Phenacite connects to the ascended masters and angelic beings.

WORKING WITH THE CHAKRAS

There is much discussion about the lower chakras being balanced for optimal emotional equilibrium, but we can't overlook the importance of keeping the upper energy centers in good working order as well. Phenacite is an unparalleled tool for opening and connecting the third eye and crown chakras. When we tap into our seat of our intuition—ajna, our third eye—we can learn to receive and trust messages from the universe. We begin to assimilate that intuitiveness into our lives, which in turn has a positive effect on opening the crown chakra, sahasrara. These two, in conjunction, will allow us to make real progress on our spiritual journey.

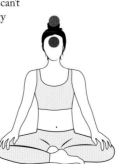

As a Pairing

Pair the otherworldly energy of phenacite with **BLACK TOURMALINE** to keep yourself grounded during spiritual journeying. Combining it with **CHRYSOPRASE** brings immense heart-healing energy, while pairing with **SELENITE** or **HERKIMER DIAMOND** enhances the high vibrations and crown chakra energy. Pair high-vibration phenacite with **GRANDIDIERITE** for a powerful combination of energies.

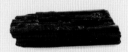

BLACK TOURMALINE

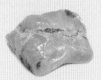

CHRYSOPRASE

SELENITE

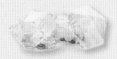

HERKIMER DIAMOND

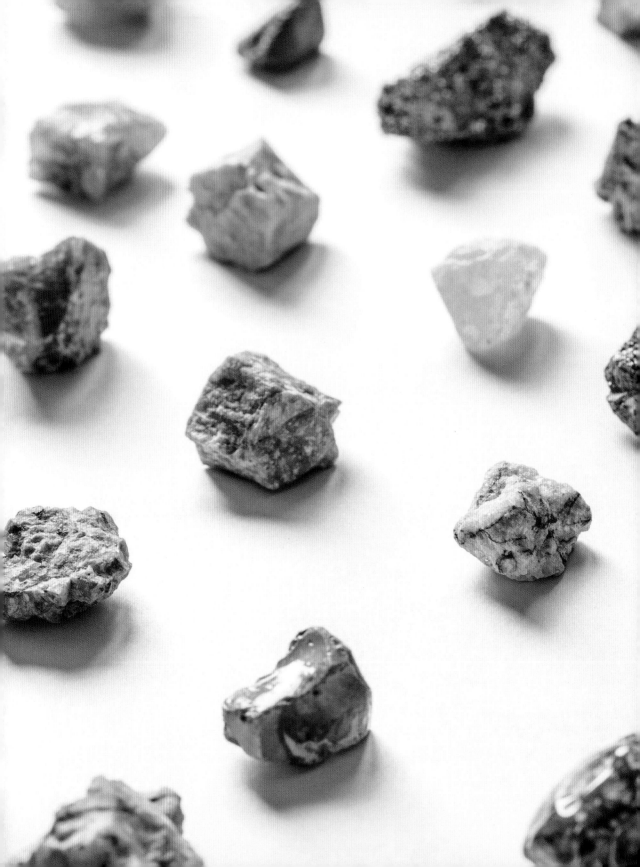

Illustrated Glossary

We may feel an instant pull toward a particular crystal—in fact, it's often said that you don't choose a crystal, but it chooses you. Other stones may reveal their significance to us more slowly over time, as we deepen our connection with them. This section provides guidance on the different ways you can use to choose which stones to work with. It also reveals the stones that are associated with the month of your birth and your star sign. In addition, you will learn how to care for your stones and use them in healing, whether singly, in pairings, or in crystal grids.

CHOOSING YOUR CRYSTAL

There are a number of methods for choosing a personal stone. You can use the
Western system as a guide or you may opt instead for an intuitive approach.
All the methods are outlined in the next few pages.

WESTERN SYSTEMS

In the West, as early as the fifth century AD, writers linked the twelve stones that
adorned the breastplate of the biblical Hebrew high priest to the twelve signs of
the zodiac. But it was not until 1912, at a meeting of the Jewelers of America, that
a consensus was reached as to an agreed pairing of birthstones with the months of
the year and the signs of the zodiac. Over the last century, this list has been updated
to include modern and often less expensive stones. Other jewellery organisations
have provided alternative lists, which allows for greater personal choice. The below
list is a mix of traditional birthstones and alternative birthstones.

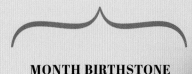

MONTH BIRTHSTONE

January > Garnet

February > Amethyst

March > Bloodstone, Aquamarine

April > Diamond, Herkimer Diamond,
Clear Quartz

May > Emerald

June > Pearl, Moonstone, Alexandrite

July > Ruby

August > Peridot, Spinel, Sardonyx

September > Sapphire, Lapis Lazuli

October > Opal, Tourmaline

November > Yellow Topaz, Citrine

December > Blue Topaz, Turquoise, Zircon,
Tanzanite, Lapis Lazuli

STAR SIGN CRYSTALS

If your birthstone does not appeal to you, then you may prefer to pick stones associated with your star sign.

♈	**Aries**	Mar 21–Apr 19	Herkimer Diamond, Aquamarine, Hematite, Dravite, Clear Quartz, Vanadinite, Red Coral
♉	**Taurus**	Apr 20–May 20	Emerald, Morganite, Chrysopase, Moldavite, Rose Quartz, Jade, Selenite, Clear Quartz, Sapphire
♊	**Gemini**	May 21–Jun 20	Moonstone, Emerald, Chrysoprase, Tiger's Eye, Phenacite, Sapphire
♋	**Cancer**	Jun 21–Jul 22	Ruby, Shungite, Grandidierite, Morganite, Honey Calcite
♌	**Leo**	Jul 23 –Aug 22	Peridot, Black Onyx, Pyrite, Sunstone, Amber
♍	**Virgo**	Aug 23–Sep 22	Emerald, Moss Agate, Carnelian, Vanadinite, Sapphire
♎	**Libra**	Sep 23–Oct 22	Opal, Black Tourmaline, Lepidolite, Phenacite, Jade, Sunstone, Sapphire
♏	**Scorpio**	Oct 23–Nov 21	Topaz, Rhodochrosite, Smoky Quartz, Grandidierite, Kunzite, Citrine, Charoite, Red Coral
♐	**Sagittarius**	Nov 22–Dec 21	Charoite, Turquoise, Blue Topaz, K2 Jasper, Lapis Lazuli
♑	**Capricorn**	Dec 22–Jan 19	Garnet, Malachite, Black Tourmaline, Fluorite, Sapphire
♒	**Aquarius**	Jan 20–Feb 18	Amethyst, Aquamarine, Hematite, Lithium Quartz, Amber, Sapphire
♓	**Pisces**	Feb 19–Mar 20	Aquamarine, Fluorite, Grandidierite, Labradorite, Larimar

INTUITIVE APPROACHES TO CHOOSING STONES

You may wish to choose a stone to work with by sight, instinct after having undertaken research, or even randomly. What's important is to choose each stone with care and reverence.

COLOR

One of the greatest attractions of a crystal is its color. Use the following method to select personal stones that will help you over longer periods of time, or for particular purposes.

1   Have before you a selection of stones. Close your eyes and allow your breathing to settle.

2   Have the intention that, when you open your eyes, you will be drawn to a crystal that is appropriate as your personal stone.

3   Open your eyes and pay attention to where they come to rest. The crystal upon which your gaze has fallen can become your personal stone.

PROPERTIES

Reading about different crystals is a good way to get an overall assessment of how each one is commonly perceived by those who have studied their powers. Some crystals will seem to match your personality quite closely; these would make useful personal stones.

RANDOM SELECTION

A random choice of a personal stone can be ideal for choosing a stone for the day. The following method works particularly well.

1   Place all your stones inside a cloth bag.

2   Relax and slow down your breathing.

3   Have in your mind a clear intention to find a personal stone for that day.

4   Dip your hand into the bag and pull out one stone.

5   Look up the properties of the stone you have chosen using this book, and consider performing the associated daily ritual.

HOW TO CONNECT
WITH ANGELS AND DEITIES

Crystals have been associated with divine beings in almost every culture over the millennia. They feature in countless myths and rituals, and many were used as amulets and/or offerings to the gods. If you are inspired by a particular deity or wish to draw on the qualities that they represent, then this can be another good way to choose a crystal to work with. Look at the list on these pages, and then go to the relevant page of the directory to discover more about the connection between the divine being and the associated crystal. You may like to hold the crystal you have chosen and bring the deity to mind, while asking for their assistance and guidance.

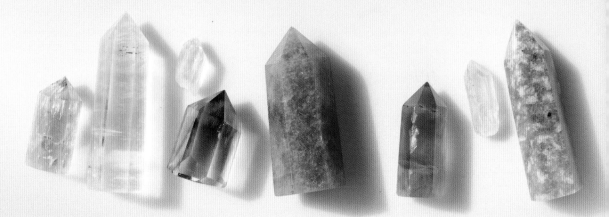

Aphrodite	Greek goddess of love and beauty	*Love, Self-care, Vitality*	Emerald, Rose Quartz
Apollo	Greek and Roman god of sun and prophecy	*Joy, Confidence*	Topaz, Sapphire
Archangel Raphael	An archangel of healing	*Divine Protection, Healing*	Emerald
Arianrhod	Welsh goddess of the moon and northern lights	*Transformation, Fertility, Spirituality*	Labradorite
Astarte	Ancient warrior goddess of love and fertility	*Love, Abundance*	Morganite
Athena	Greek goddess of wisdom and war	*Wisdom, Bravery*	K2 Jasper
Chalchiuhtlicue	Aztec goddess of fertility, streams, rivers, and lakes	*Fertility, Abundance*	Jade

Demeter	Greek goddess of harvest and agriculture	*Generosity, Kindness*	Citrine
Gaia	Mother Earth—a Greek primordial deity	*Wholeness, Balance*	Moldavite, Chrysoprase, Moss Agate
Ganesh	Hindu god of beginnings and good fortune	*Good Fortune, Intuition*	Moonstone
Guan Yin	Chinese goddess of mercy and unconditional love	*Compassion, Forgiveness*	Aquamarine, Rhodochrosite
Hathor	Egyptian sky goddess of love and fertility	*Feminine Wisdom, Affirmation*	Turquoise, Malachite
Inanna	Sumerian goddess of love, war, and the underworld	*Love, Wisdom*	Lapis Lazuli
Isis	Egyptian goddess of the moon, life, and magic	*Transitions, Change*	Rose Quartz, Carnelian
Krishna	Hindu god of compassion, tenderness, and love	*Transcendence, Love*	Ruby, Pearl
Kundalini	Hindu goddess of life-force energy	*Creative Power, Feminine Energy*	Clear Quartz
Manat	Pre-Islamic Arabian goddess of fate, fortune, time, and destinies	*Acceptance, Endurance*	Black Tourmaline
Mars	Roman god of war and an agricultural guardian	*Protection, Courage*	Hematite, Shungite
Pele	Hawaiian god of volcanoes and fire	*Empowerment, Abundance*	Peridot
Persephone	Greek goddess and queen of the underworld and spring	*Regeneration, New Beginnings*	Garnet, Pyrite
Ra	Egyptian god of the sun	*Creation, Leadership*	Sunstone
Selene	Greek goddess of the moon	*Purity, Gentleness, Calm*	Selenite
Vac	Hindu goddess of speech and truth	*Voicing Needs, Goal-setting, Clarity*	Fluorite, Charoite
Vanadis (Freyja)	Norse goddess of fertility and beauty	*Love, Witchcraft*	Vanadinite
Venus	Roman goddess of love, sex, beauty, and fertility	*Love, Healing*	Lepidolite, Jade, Emerald, Chrysoprase, Kunzite

REIKI

Reiki is Japanese for "universal life energy," and it is the word used to describe a system of natural healing that involves the laying of hands to facilitate the flow of energy around the "receiver." The "sender" gently places their hands on or just above different areas of the client's body. The energy flows from the palms of the hands of the sender into the receiver, who may experience sensations of heat or tingling and a deep sense of relaxation.

Although Reiki is a standalone technique, many senders like to incorporate crystals into their healing work. Stones can be placed on the chakras, or on other parts of the body, in order to focus the healing on a particular area. They can also be placed around the person or in a grid nearby (see page 121 for more on crystal grids). Since offering Reiki requires focus, some practitioners like to meditate with crystals beforehand or simply to have a favorite crystal on their person or in the room. You'll find ideas for using crystals with Reiki in the directory entries, but, as always, be guided by your intuition and innate knowledge.

CHAKRAS

The placing of crystals on and around the body for healing purposes seems to be an amalgamation of ideas from different traditions. Knowledge from India on the subtle anatomy of the human body—particularly the seven main chakra centers—has been combined with color therapy theories that connect parts of the body with each of the colors of the rainbow spectrum.

The driving principle behind chakra healing is to maintain a free flow of energy throughout the body, and you can use crystals to aid this process. The seven chakras used for healing represent the body's energy centers, and any blockages or other problems with the relevant part of the body can lead to illness or spiritual or emotional discomfort. Each chakra has specific healing powers, and focusing on them can help bring relief. Each of the chakras is also associated with a specific color, and choosing crystals of the relevant color to place on a chakra can energize it, so intensifying the healing effect.

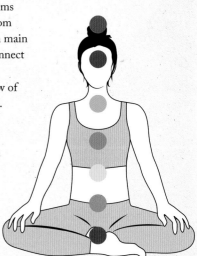

At the very top of the body, the **crown chakra** (*sahasrara*) acts as a channel for the entrance of universal energies into the body and mind, and defines, sustains, and energizes the whole chakra system. The crown chakra is the key to spiritual connections and pure happiness.

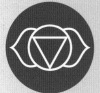

The **third eye chakra** (*ajna*) influences the functioning of the mind, helping with physical coordination, dexterity, balance, and learning skills, as well as encouraging orderliness and an increased structure in your affairs. It also drives your ability to appreciate the big picture with imagination and wisdom, and will help you to think clearly and make good decisions.

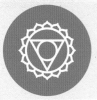

Energizing the **throat chakra** (*vishuddha*) can help to encourage creative expression and communication skills. Relieving imbalances in this area will help to promote good communication and expression, and aid in the acceptance of the truth and your own and other people's feelings.

The physical heart and the **heart chakra** (*anahata*) are the centers of the physical and subtle bodies, and have an important effect on the whole body. If the heart is truly in balance, everything else follows naturally. A sense of harmony, ease, self-confidence, and clarity of mind are engendered, and these qualities naturally enhance your relationships with others.

The **solar plexus chakra** (*manipura*) relates to the maintenance of your personal energy levels, helping you to remain in control and confident. Problems with this chakra can lead to reduced self-worth, lack of confidence, and low self-esteem.

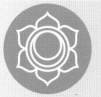

The **sacral chakra** (*svadhisthana*) controls your ability to accept others and new experiences, including pleasure and sexuality. Stress and trauma tend to become lodged here, so crystals that can restore balance or energize this chakra can help to heal anxiety, release stress, and enable you to enjoy life more fully.

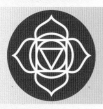

Many crystals, when placed on the **root chakra** (*muladhara*), will help to "ground" someone who is confused, overstimulated, or distracted by too many different demands or activities, helping them to focus on what is important. The root chakra is also the source of our life force, and working with it can help to integrate spiritual qualities into your everyday life.

SETTING THE SCENE

Before you work with crystals, they need to be cleansed to ensure they are free of all outside influences and energies. Most hard crystals can be safely washed in slightly soapy water. Softer crystals may become damaged by washing, and so other methods of cleansing will be necessary. Below are a range of alternatives to cleansing with soap and water.

SOUND

An easy cleansing method involves the use of bells, hand cymbals, or singing bowls. Sound of a fine quality and piercing resonance will help the crystals to release any negative energy. If you are placing crystals in a singing bowl, put a small piece of fabric in the bottom to help keep them from rattling together.

INCENSE

Incense is an easy and effective cleansing method. Each stone can be passed through the incense smoke several times. Traditional purifying incenses, such as sandalwood, frankincense, palo santo, and pine, are popular, as are the white sage and cedars generally used by Native Americans in order to cleanse their ritual spaces. Another option is to tie dried lavender stalks together and burn them, as these give off a pleasing aromatic smoke. The burning of bay leaves creates a pungent cleansing smoke.

SALT

It is inadvisable to use salted water for cleansing, as the salt crystals lodge in the crevices of the crystals being cleansed and this can dull some surfaces. Dry sea salt can, however, be used; simply pile it onto the crystals to be cleansed and leave for twenty-four hours. (Remember, don't use the salt for cooking afterward!)

SUNLIGHT

Crystals pick up negative influences over time, so it is helpful to "recharge" them regularly. Leave your stone in direct sunlight for a few hours, and then feel its warmth and renewed sense of power.

MOONLIGHT

Moonlight imbues crystals with a more subtle energy than sunlight—one that can be particularly helpful in times when introspection and calm is needed. Wait until a full moon and then place the crystal in a safe, open place and leave it overnight.

SELENITE

Selenite is a powerful crystal that can be used to cleanse and charge another crystal. Try to keep the two crystals in contact with each other, and choose a space that you can leave undisturbed for twenty-four hours. Learn more about this crystal on pages 108–109.

EARTH

You can bury your crystal in soil to cleanse and recharge it with earth energy. This can be done in your backyard or in a pot or jar.

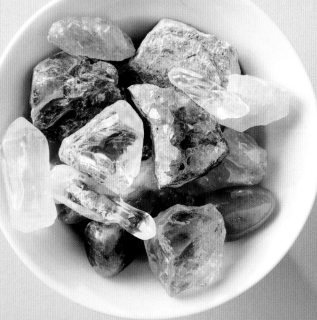

CRYSTAL GRIDS

Crystal grids are a way of setting out crystals in a pattern that has been carefully selected for a specific purpose. Grids bring together crystal energy, sacred shapes, and focused intention: a powerful triumvirate in which every element is working toward a single goal or wish. Grids are powerful tools that you can use for the manifestation of dreams, for healing, or to ease transition.

How to build a crystal grid

1. Set your intention
This is the single most important thing you can do to manifest your dreams and create change in your life.

2. Choose your grid
There are two methods for choosing a grid. Either choose the grid suggested with the crystal of your choice or look at the shapes and see which one you are most drawn to. Then read the intentions associated with each pattern and check that it aligns with your goal or wish. You can draw your grid on a piece of paper, or keep this book with you and use it as a guide to how to lay out your stones.

3. Select your stones
Choose stones that represent your intention for the grid. You'll need a single large stone (the "focus stone") and two groups of smaller stones.

4. Choose a place
Decide where you are going to lay out your grid. Clear the space and sit quietly for a short period before you begin.

5. Set your grid
Carefully lay out your stones in your chosen grid.

Three types of stones

♦ **Focus stone:** Found most often at the center of a grid, the focus stone channels and gathers the creative power of the universe to your grid, before sending it along an energetic pathway toward the way and desire stones. While any type of crystal will work, the focus stone will usually be a larger stone, such as a cluster, point, or carved shape. If you are unsure which crystal to use, a clear quartz point or cluster is always a safe bet as a focus stone.

♦ **Way stone:** Most often consisting of tumbled stones or points that are arranged in the area immediately surrounding the focus stone, the way stones create a pathway toward your end result. When choosing your way stone, ask yourself, "How am I going to get there?" Will it be by way of courage? Clear communication? Self-love? Knowing the answers will help you to choose the most useful way stones.

♦ **Desire stone:** Typically consisting of tumbled stones or points arranged around the outer edges of your grid, the desire stone is the one most closely associated with your goal. When choosing your desire stone, simply ask yourself, "What do I desire?" Is it financial wealth? Self-confidence? Romance? The answer will help you to decide on the perfect fit for your desire stone.

THE GRIDS

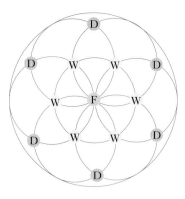

Seed of Life

Choose this grid to:

- Manifest dreams and goals
- See any task or project through to completion
- Maintain energy and stamina
- Build new habits and strengthen willpower
- Enhance creativity
- Attract good luck and abundance

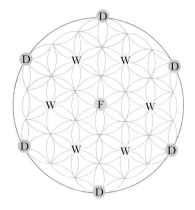

Flower of Life

Choose this grid to:

- Promote knowledge and inner awareness
- Increase confidence and self-esteem
- Manifest goals and desires
- Restore harmony and balance
- Enhance creativity
- Attract wealth and abundance

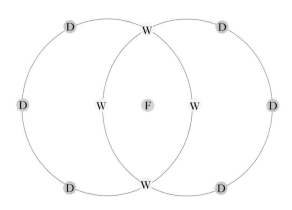

Vesica Piscis

Choose this grid to:

- Improve relationships
- Inspire harmony and balance
- Promote understanding
- Connect with others and your higher self
- Promote rebirth and transformation

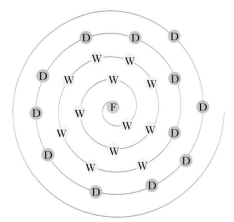

Spiral

Choose this grid to:

- Improve health
- Enhance stamina and focus
- Provide a sense of grounding
- Expand knowledge and heighten consciousness
- Support personal growth of any kind

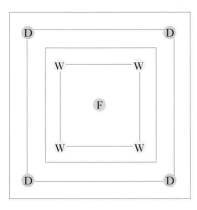

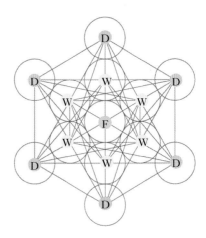

Square

Choose this grid to:

– Set and maintain personal boundaries
– Inspire a sense of safety and protection
– Build on goals and dreams
– Improve self-confidence
– Enhance feelings of stability and security

Metatron's Cube

Choose this grid to:

– Replace negative thoughts with
  positive ones
– Promote balance
– Manifest feelings of happiness
  and patience

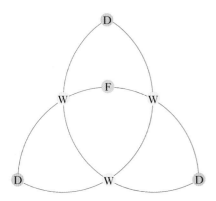

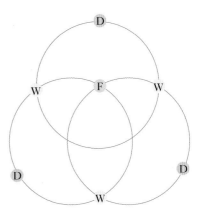

Tripod of Life

Choose this grid to:

– Start a family
– Bring a new project or venture to life
– Boost creativity
– Build an intense romantic connection
– Begin a new journey of any kind

Borromean Rings

Choose this grid to:

– Offer support in matters related to
  friendships, work, or family
– Inspire teamwork and cooperation
– Alleviate tension
– Deepen all forms of connection
– Invoke miracles of all kinds

INDEX

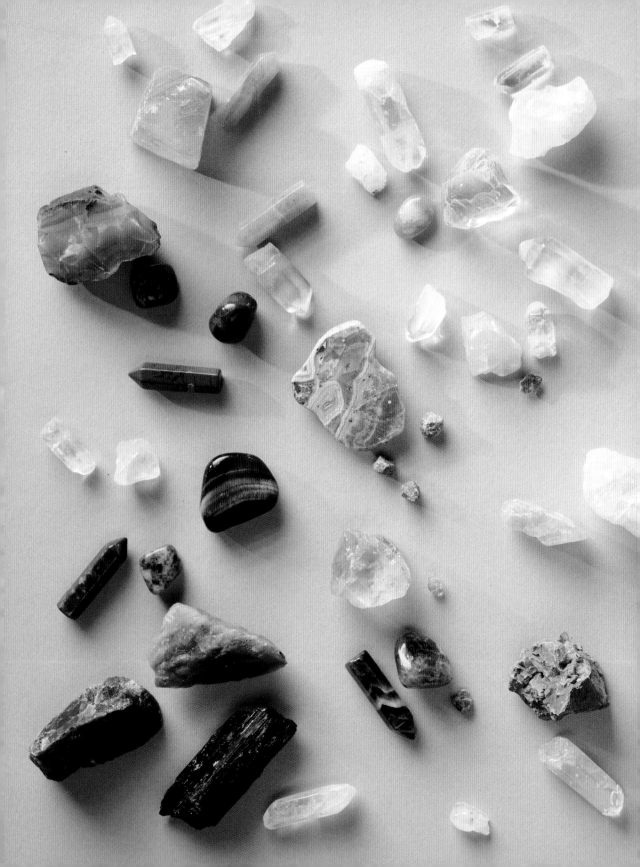

RESOURCES

Websites
Crystal Vaults
www.crystalvaults.com
Shop for crystals by color, shape, or type, and enjoy some free
online crystal guides.

Healing Crystals
www.healingcrystals.com
Providing affordable and quality crystals worldwide.

Hibiscus Moon Crystal Academy
www.hibiscusmooncrystalacademy.com
A globally accredited crystal course provider.

Sage Goddess
www.sagegoddess.com
Shop for a wide array of crystals and other sacred tools.

Sea Ox Designs
www.seaoxdesigns.com
Shop for crystals, earring, rings, home decor, and more.

Minerals.net
Minerals.net
Mineral and gemstone guide, community, gallery, and research.

Books
Book of Stones by Robert Simmons and Naisha Ahsian
Crystal Bible by Judy Hall

ACKNOWLEDGMENTS

For Charlie and Wolffe, my most precious gems.

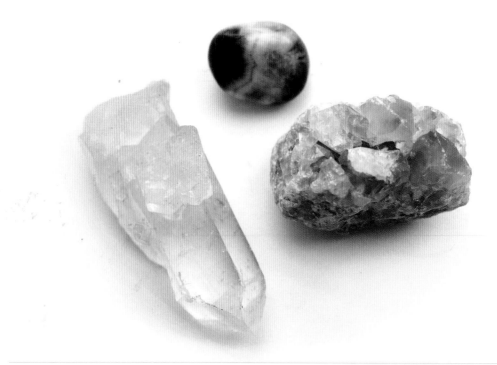

CREDITS

Quarto would like to thank the following Shutterstock contributors for supplying images for inclusion in this book:

Albert Russ/Shutterstock.com; Alena Solonshchikova/Shutterstock.com; Alex Coan/Shutterstock.com; Alexander Hoffmann/Shutterstock.com; Anastasia Bulanova/Shutterstock.com; annetipodees/Shutterstock.com; Anno/Shutterstock.com; Art Stocker/Shutterstock.com; Arthur Balitskii/Shutterstock.com; Bjoern Wylezich/Shutterstock.com; Bodor Tivadar/Shutterstock.com; Christy Liem/Shutterstock.com; Cute art/Shutterstock.com; eloresnorwood/Shutterstock.com; Epitavi/Shutterstock.com; Ilizia/Shutterstock.com; Imfoto/Shutterstock.com; KrimKate/Shutterstock.com; La corneja artesana/Shutterstock.com; mahirart/Shutterstock.com; Masianya/Shutterstock.com; michal812/Shutterstock.com; Minakryn Ruslan/Shutterstock.com; MXW Stock/Shutterstock.com; Napoleonka/Shutterstock.com; Natalie Dvorackova/Shutterstock.com; Neirfy/Shutterstock.com; New Africa/Shutterstock.com; Nikki Zalewski/Shutterstock.com; olpo/Shutterstock.com; photo-world/Shutterstock.com; Polnocha/Shutterstock.com; Reload Design/Shutterstock.com; RHJPhtotos/Shutterstock.com; Roy Palmer/Shutterstock.com; Semiglass/Shutterstock.com; Sentelia/Shutterstock.com; Tamara Kulikova/Shutterstock.com; Travelling Jack/Shutterstock.com; Tycson1/Shutterstock.com; vvoe/Shutterstock.com; Wirestock Creators/Shutterstock.com.